Croner's PREGNANCY AND MATERNITY RIGHTS

Emma Cowell,
Anthony Korn
and
Paul Nicholls
of
Dibb Lupton Broomhead

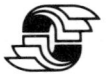

CRONER PUBLICATIONS LIMITED

Croner House, London Road
Kingston upon Thames
Surrey KT2 6SR
Tel: 081-547 3333

Copyright © Croner Publications Ltd
First published 1993
Second edition 1994

Published by
Croner Publications Ltd,
Croner House,
London Road,
Kingston upon Thames,
Surrey KT2 6SR
Tel: 081-547 3333

All rights reserved.
No part of this publication may be reproduced,
stored in a retrieval system, or transmitted in any form or by
any means, electronic, mechanical, photocopying, recording,
or otherwise without the prior permission of
Croner Publications Ltd.

While every care has been taken
in the writing and editing of this book,
readers should be aware that only Acts of Parliament
and Statutory Instruments have the force of law
and that only the courts can authoritatively
interpret the law.

British Library Cataloguing in Publication Data
A CIP Catalogue Record for this book
is available from the British Library

ISBN: 1 85524 283 4

Typeset by Concept Communications Ltd, Crayford, Kent
Printed by Whitstable Litho Ltd, Whitstable, Kent

Contents

Introduction 1

1 Ante-natal Care 3

Introduction
What is Ante-natal Care?
The Statutory Right to Time Off Work
Abuse of the Right
Contractual Rights
Remedies
Infertility Treatment
Questions and Answers

2 Sex Discrimination and Pregnancy 19

Introduction
The Sex Discrimination Act 1975
Case Law
The "Equal Treatment Directive"
European Community Approach
The English "Comparative" Approach
Questions and Answers

3 Maternity Leave and the Right to Return to Work 33

Introduction
The New Right to Short-term Maternity Leave
The Statutory Maternity Leave Period
Long-term Maternity Leave
The Right to Return to Work
Suspension Rights

Maternity Dismissals
　　　Automatic Right to Written Reasons
　　　　　for Dismissal
　　　Questions and Answers

4 Redundancy   69

　　　Introduction
　　　Suitable Alternative Vacancy
　　　Implementing Redundancies
　　　Notice Payments
　　　Repayment of Redundancy Monies
　　　Questions and Answers

5 Maternity Pay   79

　　　Introduction
　　　Maternity Allowance
　　　Statutory Maternity Pay
　　　Calculating the Qualifying Week
　　　Agency Workers
　　　Seasonal or Regular Casual Workers
　　　Change of Employer
　　　Average Weekly Earnings
　　　Notification of Maternity Absence
　　　Rates of SMP
　　　The Maternity Pay Period
　　　Events which may Disentitle the
　　　　　Employee from SMP
　　　Payment and Administration of
　　　　　SMP
　　　Mistakes
　　　Records
　　　Insolvency of Employer
　　　Different Types of Pregnancy
　　　Contractual Maternity Pay
　　　Questions and Answers

6	**Disputes and Appeals**	113

    Internal Grievance Procedure
    A Written Statement
    Application to an Adjudication Officer
    Appeal Against an Adjudication
        Officer's Decision
    Further Appeal
    Disputes Reserved for The Secretary
        of State
    Review as Opposed to Appeal
    Enforcement of Formal Decisions
    Questions and Answers

7	**Health and Safety**	125

    Pregnant Workers Directive
    TURERA 1993 Provisions
    Display Screen Equipment
    Questions and Answers

Glossary	137
Further Information	139
Index	143

Introduction

Ever since it was first introduced in the mid 1970s, the right to maternity leave and maternity pay has caused difficulties for employers. The message that women are entitled to leave is one that has been very difficult to convey to line managers. Personnel professionals are frequently faced with trying to recover a situation where a line manager has effectively dismissed a pregnant employee by telling her that there will be no job for her to return to.

Statistically, the number of women who return to work has been growing steadily. Whereas, not many years ago, approximately only one in three women returned to work, it is now more than one in two.

There is now the added complication of the overlay of the EC Pregnant Workers Directive and the Government's implementation, which means that there will be two separate schemes running in tandem. The first will give every woman the right to return to work after 14 weeks' maternity leave, regardless of the length of her service, but the old extended leave (11 weeks ante-natal, 29 post-natal) will still continue to operate for women with more than two years' service.

The Government introduced the legislation in relation to the new 14 weeks' maternity leave in the Trade Union Reform and Employment Rights Act 1993 which will effect women whose EWC falls on or after the 16 October 1994. The Directive also requires them to make arrangements for women to receive maternity pay of not less than the minimum statutory sick pay during the period of their maternity leave.

This pocket book is designed to help employers through the legalistic maze connected with maternity rights. It is designed to help ensure that the right benefits and entitlements are given to staff and that employers do not fall unawares into a breach of any of the relevant legislation. Currently, women with less than 26 weeks' service will not be entitled to any maternity pay, but may be entitled to maternity allowance, and so will either have to take an unpaid period of leave, or otherwise receive a discretionary payment. At the same time, employers should ensure that staff with less than 26 weeks' service taking sick leave are treated in the same way.

The book is arranged to follow the progress of the pregnancy. First we deal with the right to ante-natal time off work, then sex discrimination and pregnancy, followed by the right to maternity leave and the right to return to work. We cover the issue of maternity pay and the administration of a maternity pay scheme. In this latter regard, the proposals to require employers to make a contribution to the maternity pay scheme have been finalised. It is simply the question that the level of recovery has been reduced for the employer.

We have also included a questions and answers section at the end of each chapter, which we very much hope will be of value.

1 Ante-natal Care

Introduction

All employees, regardless of their length of service or hours of service, have the right to reasonable time off work for ante-natal care. The right to time off is on full pay and the employee can seek compensation from the employer if she is refused time off or is not paid sufficiently or at all for the time off.

The right to paid time off for ante-natal care was introduced by the Employment Act 1980 and was incorporated into the Employment Protection (Consolidation) Act 1978 (EP(C)A). The right was primarily introduced as a response to the medical profession progressively emphasising the importance of ante-natal treatment and in order to encourage pregnant employees to attend ante-natal clinics without the threat of loss of pay. Until the Trade Union Reform and Employment Rights Act 1993 (TURERA 1993) most of a pregnant employee's statutory rights, as detailed in the EP(C)A, were subject to an employee having two years' continuous service. The right to paid time off for ante-natal care was the notable exception since it is the right of all employees irrespective of their length of service. Ante-natal care should be distinguished from sickness during maternity and actual maternity leave, both of which are covered later.

What is Ante-natal Care?

The term primarily refers to the period before a pregnant woman gives birth. However, employers may find themselves faced with an employee requesting time off before actually becoming pregnant, for example, for attendance at a hospital or clinic for infertility treatment. We shall come back to the issue of infertility treatment later in this chapter.

Having set out the right in s.31A, the Act does not define "ante-natal care" other than by stating that it must be on the advice of a registered medical practitioner, midwife or health visitor. It would in fact be very difficult categorically to define what is meant by "ante-natal care" since obviously it may vary depending upon the medical condition and the general state of health of the particular employee concerned.

It is, however, possible to give general guidelines in terms of what medical advisors often describe as the "standard" ante-natal clinic visits. As a general rule, most women make their first visit to the ante-natal clinic somewhere between the eighth and 12th week of pregnancy and then, subject to the individual's medical condition, visits are generally made thereafter on a monthly basis. In the last few months of the pregnancy it is thought advisable for the pregnant woman to attend the clinic every few weeks and during the final stages of pregnancy a weekly visit is recommended. These "standard" visits will undoubtedly fall within the definition of "ante-natal care".

The employee's right as regards time off work to attend relaxation classes is less clear cut, although the tribunal held in *Gregory v Tudsbury (1982) IRLR 267* that the term ante-natal care was in fact wide enough to include attendance at relaxation classes. At the same time, however, if the employee is unable to show the employer that she is attending the relaxation classes on the recommendation of her medical advisors, she may find that she is refused paid time off for their attendance. Therefore, if she is able to provide a statement from her medical advisors emphasising the importance of her attendance at such classes as part of her ante-natal treatment, an employer may take the view that she should be allowed paid time off to attend them.

The question has arisen as to whether an appointment made by an employee to see her doctor to ascertain whether or not she is pregnant would be included within the definition of ante-natal care. If the employee in fact turns out to be pregnant then she has simply received "ante-natal care". However, on a strict interpretation of the Act, an employee who is told that she is not pregnant does not enjoy this statutory right.

The Statutory Right to Time Off Work

Qualification

Paid time off for ante-natal care is a right to which all pregnant employees are entitled by statute. The right is not subject to the employee satisfying a condition of continuous employment nor is there a minimum number of hours worked requirement.

For paid time off for attendance at the first ante-natal appointment the employee needs to satisfy the following:

- the employee must be pregnant, and
- an appointment must have been made to receive ante-natal care on the advice of a registered medical practitioner, registered midwife or registered health visitor — s.31A(1).

For attendance at subsequent appointments, the employee may be required to produce for the employer's inspection:

- a certificate from a registered medical practitioner, registered midwife or registered health visitor stating that the employee is pregnant, and
- an appointment card or some other document showing that the appointment has been made — s.31A(2).

Therefore, if an employee fails to provide the employer with the above on request, then the employer is not required to permit the employee to take paid time off to keep an appointment.

How Much Time Off?

The right to time off during working hours is qualified by a condition of reasonableness. Section 31A specifically states that the employee has "the right not to be unreasonably refused time off during her working hours".

The wording anticipates certain instances when it would be reasonable for the employer to refuse to give a pregnant employee paid time off, but the law is not particularly helpful here since no guidance is given as to how one should determine what is "reasonable" or "unreasonable". As a general rule, tribunals are reluctant to find that a refusal is reasonable when medical advisors have recommended that an appointment be made. In *Gregory v Tudsbury (1982) IRLR 267*, the tribunal suggested that "there may be circumstances where it may be reasonable for an employer to refuse an employee time off if it is reasonable in the circumstances that the employee can make arrangements outside normal working hours". The tribunal did not provide examples of situations which would justify a reasonable refusal on behalf of the employer but simply stated that the decision should be made on the merits of each individual case. For example, part-time staff and shift workers may be included in this category and employers may be able to argue that for attendance at non-urgent ante-natal classes and/or relaxation classes, an employer may not be acting unreasonably in refusing paid time off, if an employee could reasonably arrange the appointments outside her normal working hours. If an employee refuses to co-operate with such a request without good reason it may be perfectly within the employer's right to refuse her paid time off. Of course, in practice the timing of appointments is generally outside the individual's control and so it may not always be possible for the employee to arrange an appointment outside her normal working hours. An employee is expected to comply with such a request as far as possible and if unable to do so she should be able to justify this to her employer.

When a pregnancy is not "standard" and visits to the ante-natal clinic are unusually frequent, the employer may face real difficulties covering the absent employee's work. In addition, the actual length of absence for attendance at the appointment may also be a problem for the employer. For example, the particular clinic being visited may be located a substantial way from the place of employment, which adds to the length of time the employee is actually absent from the workplace. In essence, what is reasonable time off for one pregnant employee may not be reasonable time off for another. The needs of the pregnant employee should be weighed against the needs of the company, but it is for the employer to show that he or she has acted reasonably. The burden of proof is upon the employer in this instance in any proceedings upon the matter.

The Right to Time Off During Working Hours

The employee's right is to time off "during the employee's working hours". Therefore, it would not be reasonable for the employer to avoid this by, for example, requiring the employee to make up her lost time by rearranging her working hours. In the case of *Edgar v Giorgione Inns Ltd COIT 1803/13*, their reason for not paying the employee for her time off was that she should either have rearranged her appointments for outside office hours or at least have worked on Sundays to make up for the lost time. The tribunal stated that to the contrary: "There is no provision in the Act to the effect that [the employee] has to reorganise her working hours to make up for lost hours by working at weekends or at some other time."

Employee Must Provide Evidence of the Appointment

An employer is not required to give an employee paid time off to attend an ante-natal appointment if the employee fails to comply with s.31A(2) of the EP(C)A. This subsection provides that an employer shall not be required to permit an employee to take time off to attend an appointment unless she complies with an employer's request to produce a certificate of pregnancy from either a registered medical practitioner, a registered midwife or a registered health visitor and an appointment card or such other documentation evidencing that an appointment has been made. This subsection does not apply where the appointment is the employee's first appointment for which permission has been sought in accordance with subsection (1). Of course, the requirement to produce the certificate and appointment card is only necessary where the employer has actually specifically asked to see them. Consequently, in the case of *Edgar v Giorgione Inns Ltd COIT 1803/13*, the employers relied on the fact that the employee had failed to show her appointment cards. However, it was held that their non-production was wholly irrelevant since the employer had never actually requested to see them.

Pay Entitlement

Section 31A(4) of the EP(C)A provides that "an employee who is permitted to take time off during her working hours in accordance with subsection (1) shall be entitled to be paid remuneration by her employer for the period of absence at the appropriate hourly rate".

Consequently, an employer should never tell an employee that she can have time off but without pay.

In *Gregory v Tudsbury Ltd (1992) IRLR 267*, the employer allowed the employee time off for attendance at her ante-natal appointments, but refused to pay her for that time off on the basis that it was within the employer's rights reasonably to refuse to do so. This was held by the tribunal to be incorrect and the tribunal found that once an employer allows an employee time off they are automatically bound to pay the employee for that time off. It would have been a very different situation if the employer had simply refused to give the employee time off since it would then have been for the tribunal to decide whether or not the refusal was reasonable. If the employee is given time off, she is automatically entitled to receive payment for it and if payment is not forthcoming the employee can lodge a complaint at an industrial tribunal and receive compensation of the pay lost (see below).

The employer is obliged under the Act to pay the employee for the "time needed to keep her appointment". Of course, this could be considerably longer than the actual appointment itself when one takes into account travel time, waiting time etc. In the unreported case of *Dhamrait v United Biscuits Ltd* the industrial tribunal held that the pregnant employee was entitled to be paid for the whole of her shift even though in theory her appointment was scheduled to last only one hour. In fact, the actual appointment lasted longer than anticipated and together with the unreliable public transport to and from the office she was actually absent from the office for the whole of her shift. It was held that she was entitled to receive payment for the whole of her shift since the tribunal took the view that that was the time necessary to enable the employee to fulfil her appointment.

The entitlement is to payment at the "appropriate hourly rate". The "appropriate hourly rate" is defined as one "week's pay" divided by "the number of normal working hours in a week for that employee under the contract in force on the day when the time off is taken" — s.31A(5)(a).

The "normal working hours" and a "week's pay" are computed in accordance with Schedule 14, Part I and Part II respectively of the EP(C)A.

It is interesting to note that there is no ceiling on a "week's pay" as there is for example with redundancy payments.

The Act sets out three alternative formulae to be used to calculate the amount due and owing to the employee:

(a) Where normal working hours do not vary, the following formula is applied:

$$\frac{\text{A week's pay}}{\text{Normal working hours under the contract of employment}}$$

(b) Where the number of hours worked varies from week to week the following formula is applied:

$$\frac{\text{A week's pay}}{\text{Average normal working hours}}$$

The average is calculated by dividing by 12 the total number of the employee's normal working hours during the 12 weeks immediately prior to the week in which the appointment occurred.

The "pay week" for employees who are paid on a weekly basis ends with the day on which they are actually paid and for other employees the "pay week" ends on Saturday.

(c) Where an employee's normal working hours vary as in (b) above, but the employee has not worked for 12 weeks, the employee has not been employed for long enough for the calculation set out in (b) above to be made and the following formula is applied:

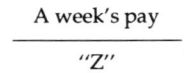

$$\frac{\text{A week's pay}}{\text{"Z"}}$$

"Z" represents an average number of normal working hours in a week which the employee could reasonably have expected to have worked under her contract of employment or the average number of hours worked by comparable employees.

Abuse of the Right

At the most basic level the employer could allow the employee to take the time off but refuse to pay and leave it to the employee to take proceedings against him or her in the industrial tribunal. She may not make any claim if she is aware that her conduct has not been reasonable and, apart from the cost of the proceedings and possible adverse publicity, the worst that could happen to the employer is that the employee would be awarded the lost pay. There are dangers in actually refusing to allow her to take the time off. She might complain of constructive dismissal. If the tribunal could properly take the view that she was protected by s.31A of the Act her claim would succeed. The tribunal has the power to, and probably would, order reinstatement in such a case if she wanted it, or otherwise give her compensation. If she had more than two years' service she would rely on the EP(C)A for her claim, but otherwise she would allege that the refusal to allow her time off for ante-natal care amounted to sex discrimination (see Chapter 2).

In Cases of Fraud

If the employee has fabricated a doctor's certificate or hospital appointment (or perhaps not attended the hospital appointment but spent the day shopping) this would be a matter of gross misconduct and the employee should be subjected to the organisation's disciplinary procedures in the normal way, given an opportunity to refute the allegation or otherwise explain or excuse her conduct.

In Cases of Unauthorised Absence

This would be a matter of misconduct, rather than gross misconduct. The individual should be subjected to the organisation's normal disciplinary procedures and, if appropriate, given a warning and advised that further repetition of such unauthorised absence could lead to dismissal. If there were such repetitions (two warnings would normally be appropriate) then, again subject to a disciplinary hearing, the individual could be dismissed on notice. It is important that the disciplinary hearing in every case explores fully the reason for the absence.

Contractual Rights

Some employees will also have the benefit of contractual rights in respect of time off for ante-natal care regardless of whether the time off is on the advice of medical advisors, as this is what is set out in the contract of employment, company handbook, or perhaps a union agreement. Where an employee has the contractual right to take paid time off, the employee has the option of enjoying either her contractual or her statutory entitlement. An employee does not have the right to receive both the contractual pay and the statutory pay since this would result in a double recovery by the employee for that period. If the contractual entitlement is less than the statutory then she is entitled to the benefit of the statutory scheme.

The employer's statutory liability will be discharged by the contractual agreement so long as the contractual amount is at least equal to the statutory minimum. The legislation provides the employee with a legal minimum amount of pay and the employer is not permitted to reduce the amount by entering into a contract with her for a lesser sum. The provisions contained in s.31A(4) are a means of ensuring that if there is no contractual right to remuneration then in any event the employee is guaranteed that her wage will not be reduced to take account of the time for which she is absent from the workplace to attend her appointment.

Any contractual rights in relation to this matter should obviously be set down in writing in the usual way so that employees are entirely clear as to what their rights are. If it is intended that this right should be discretionary then this should be clearly stated and, to avoid confusion or mistakes, the absolute statutory minimum entitlement (which of course is not discretionary) should be set out. An employer should be careful of unintentionally creating a precedent which future employees may try to rely upon. Custom and practice can become "contractual" in status if it becomes obvious to all that this is standard practice. To avoid situations arising and an employer unintentionally granting contractual rights, each individual case should be evidenced in writing making it clear that leave was only granted after full consideration had been given to the merits of that particular employee's case. In this way, the right is granted purely on a discretionary basis and no precedent is set which would make it difficult for the employer to refuse the same to another employee in the future.

Remedies

In accordance with s.31A(6), an employee may complain to an industrial tribunal and get compensation on either of the following two grounds:

- that her employer has unreasonably refused her time off for ante-natal care, or
- that her employer failed to pay (in whole or part) the amount due to her in accordance with s.31A(4) for the time off.

The employee must present her complaint within three months of the day of the particular appointment although the tribunal have discretion to extend the time limit for such further period as they consider reasonable if they are of the view that it was not reasonably practicable for the employee to comply with the time limit. If the tribunal takes the view that it was not reasonably practicable for the employee to have presented the complaint in time then the tribunal has to decide what would in the circumstances be a reasonable further period in which to allow her to present her complaint — s.31A(7). This is a strict test. Ignorance of her right, or misguided professional advice, are not good "excuses". Misleading advice from the tribunal itself, or illness, would be.

If the employee makes a complaint of being unreasonably refused time off, the burden is on the employer to show that the refusal was not in the circumstances unreasonable.

If the tribunal makes a finding that the employee's complaint is justified and that the employer was unreasonable then the tribunal must make a declaration to that effect.

If the complaint is that she has been unreasonably refused time off then the tribunal will, as well as making a declaration to that effect, also make an award of compensation equal to her entitlement under statute namely, "an amount equal to the remuneration to which she would have been entitled under subsection (4) if the time off had not been refused" — s.31A(8)(a). The effect of this award is that the employee is in fact paid twice for that particular period since there is no "set off" provision. The employee will have been paid her contractual pay as normal for working that period and she will also receive the additional payment of the same amount under the statutory award. This award is in effect a fine on employers to encourage their future compliance with the provision.

If the complaint is that the employer, although allowing the employee time off, refused to pay her for this time off either in whole or in part and the tribunal makes a finding in favour of the employee then the tribunal must make a declaration to that effect. In addition, the tribunal must make an order for payment to the employee in accordance with s.31(8)(b) of "the amount which it finds due to her".

The services of an ACAS conciliation officer are available under s.133(1)(a) in order to try to settle any complaint without proceeding to an industrial tribunal.

Infertility Treatment

As was briefly mentioned at the beginning of this chapter, employers may find themselves approached by an employee (either male or female) requesting time off work in order to attend an appointment for treatment for infertility. There is no equivalent right at law for an employee seeking such treatment not to be unreasonably refused paid time off for such an appointment. In addition, it is unlikely that an employee seeking such treatment would be regarded as absent from work due to sickness. If an employer is sympathetic to a particular case and agrees to give paid time off then it should be evidenced in writing and expressly stated that leave has been given at the employer's discretion on the basis of the merits of that particular case. This would keep the right on a discretionary basis. Alternatively the company handbook or contract could be amended to supply this as a discretionary right.

Although medical techniques in this field are improving all the time, the programme an individual has to go through is time-consuming and harrowing. It can be important that the individual takes time off at short notice as timing can be of the essence. It would be a good idea for the employer to ask for (or the employee to volunteer) a doctor's letter specifying exactly what is involved and how much time will be required. Refusal of such time off may lead to resignation and the prospect of a claim against the employer of constructive dismissal if over two years' service or, regardless of service, discrimination.

Once the individual on the infertility programme is actually pregnant then, by definition, she acquires the statutory protection to "reasonable time off" set out earlier in this chapter. It is likely that the requirement for time off work for ante-natal care will be very much more than is usual but that any tribunal would find such a requirement "reasonable".

Checklist: Ante-natal Care

- All pregnant employees are entitled to paid time off for ante-natal check ups — no qualifying service is required.
- Evidence may be required after the first visit.
- 8–12 weeks into pregnancy — check-ups start. Thereafter 1 per month.
- After 6–7 months of pregnancy — frequency will increase to 1 visit per fortnight.
- After 8 months of pregnancy — weekly visits to doctor likely.
- Contractual rights may also apply.
- Infertility treatment — no right to paid time off — not equivalent to sickness.

Questions and Answers

Q: Can I discipline an individual who takes time off without seeking anyone's permission?

A: *Yes. The right to time off for ante-natal care is "not to be unreasonably refused" which carries the clear indication that she must ask you for time off first. If you are to discipline such an employee you need to ensure that you follow procedures very carefully and that there was some bona fide immediate need for sick leave.*

Q: Do I have to pay the individual for the time she takes to travel to her hospital appointment as well as for the time off for the ante-natal care itself?

A: *Yes. You must pay the individual for all the reasonable time off she needs to attend the appointment including the travelling time.*

Q: Can I require the employee to provide evidence that she has an appointment?

A: *Yes. Except for the very first appointment you may require her to produce a certificate from her doctor or midwife or health visitor together with an appointment card showing that an appointment has been made for ante- natal care. For the first appointment you simply have to take her at her word. She must advise you that she is pregnant and the entitlement only arises on the basis that she is pregnant but you may feel it inappropriate to deny payment if it turns out that she is not.*

Q: What can the individual do if I refuse to pay her?

A: *She can make an application to an industrial tribunal for that payment.*

Q: What if I refuse to let her attend ante-natal classes?

A: *She could either make an application to an industrial tribunal for compensation equivalent to the earnings for the period that she would have been away on the appointment, otherwise if she had two years' service she could claim constructive dismissal in an industrial tribunal.*

Q: Can I require her to make up the time later?

A: *No you may not.*

Q: Can a male member of staff demand the right to accompany his wife to ante-natal classes?

A: *No. The qualification for this right is that the individual must "be pregnant".*

2 Sex Discrimination and Pregnancy

Introduction

Before considering in detail the Trade Union Reform and Employment Rights Act 1993 (TURERA 1993) it is important to consider the extent to which an employee who is pregnant, or wishes to take a period of maternity leave, might be able to rely on the Sex Discrimination Act 1975 and/or the Equal Treatment Directive.

The Sex Discrimination Act 1975 (SDA)

Section 6(1) and (2) of the SDA sets out the extent to which an employee is protected against sex discrimination.

- *"It is unlawful for a person, in relation to employment by him at an establishment in Great Britain, to discriminate against a woman:*

    (a) in the arrangement he makes for the purpose of determining who should be offered that employment, or

    (b) in the terms on which he offers her that employment, or

    (c) for refusing or deliberately omitting to offer her that employment".

- *"It is unlawful for a person, in the case of a woman employed by him at an establishment in Great Britain, to discriminate against her:*

> (a) *in the way he affords her access to opportunities for promotion, transfer or training, or to any other benefits, facilities or services, or by refusing or deliberately omitting to afford her access to them, or*
>
> (b) *by dismissing her, or subjecting her to any other detriment."*

Under s.1(1)(a) of the SDA, a person commits an act of direct sex discrimination against a woman if "on the grounds of her sex he treats her less favourably than he treats or would treat a man".

Many employers find it a surprising suggestion that it is unlawful sex discrimination to take adverse action against a female employee on grounds of pregnancy or pregnancy-related matters, such as maternity leave, since s.5(3) specifically states that in order to establish less favourable treatment the comparison of a male and a female "must be such that the relevant circumstances in the one case are the same, ... not materially different, in the other". The question of whether it is discrimination on grounds of sex contrary to the SDA to dismiss a woman from her employment because she is pregnant has produced interesting case law which we shall now consider.

Case Law

The first case to come before the Employment Appeal Tribunal (EAT) which raised this question was *Turley v Allders Department Stores (1980) ICR 66*. In that case the EAT ruled that such treatment could not amount to unlawful sex discrimination since discrimination by its very nature involves the treatment of a woman less favourably than a man, and since pregnancy is a condition unique to women, a man could never be compared with a pregnant woman.

Mr Justice Bristow actually said that "in order to see if she has been treated less favourably than a man, you must compare like with like, and you cannot. When she is pregnant a woman is no longer just a woman. She is a woman, as the Authorised Version accurately puts it, with child, and there is no masculine equivalent".

The result of this decision was that women who were dismissed for reasons relating to pregnancy or maternity, could not bring a claim under the SDA. However, the view of the EAT in *Turley* was not followed in the later case of *Hayes v Malleable Working Men's Club (1985) IRLR 367*. In *Hayes*, the EAT held that the *Turley* decision was "so devoid of any factual context as to be virtually academic" since the case decided whether a dismissal on grounds of pregnancy could amount to unlawful sex discrimination without actually considering the facts. The EAT preferred the minority view in *Turley* that a dismissal will normally be as a consequence of the pregnancy rather than the condition of pregnancy itself and that it would be very unusual nowadays for a dismissal to occur purely because the employee is going to have a child and for no other connected reason, such as the requirement to have time off work. The EAT concluded that *Turley* should either be distinguished in that its application should occur in very limited circumstances or that it should, in fact, be disregarded and not followed at all.

The EAT in *Hayes* stated that the correct approach was to ask the following questions.

> "Was it, for example, a mere fact of the pregnancy itself to which the Club objected or was it "more probably" the enforced period of absence from work which the baby's birth would require? If so, how long would the offending period of absence expect to last? Were male Club employees liable for other reasons (such as illness) to be away from work for an equivalent period, and (if so) how would they be treated?"

As a result of the decision in *Hayes*, a tribunal should ask itself three questions in deciding whether discrimination has occurred.

- What was the reason for the dismissal?
- What were the employer's objections to a pregnant employee?
- Would a "comparable man" be treated more favourably by not being dismissed?

This approach was held to satisfy the test set out in s.5(3) of the SDA of "relevant circumstances".

In *Fyfe v Farmer Giles Goods (Scotland) Ltd*, Ms Fyfe was dismissed after taking time off work as a result of excessive vomiting which was caused by her pregnancy. The industrial tribunal held that it was necessary for the comparison to be made between her treatment and the way the employer has treated, or would treat, a sick male employee. The industrial tribunal held that Ms Fyfe had been unlawfully discriminated against since a male employee who had been incapacitated for a similar length of time with damaged tendons in his shoulder had not been similarly dismissed.

The "Equal Treatment Directive"

The Council Directive 76/207/EEC of 9 February 1976 (the "Equal Treatment Directive") established the principle of equal treatment for men and women as regards access to employment, vocational training and promotion and working conditions. Article 2(1) of the Directive provides that "the principle of equal treatment shall mean that there will be no discrimination whatsoever on grounds of sex either directly or indirectly by reference in particular to marriage or family status". Article 5(1) provides that "the application of the principle of equal treatment with regard to working conditions, including the conditions governing dismissal, means that men and women are to be guaranteed the same conditions without discrimination on grounds of sex". Finally, Article 2(3) states that the directive "shall be without prejudice to provisions concerning the protection of women, particularly as regards pregnancy and maternity".

Directives are directly enforceable against the state, or emanations of the state and the UK court has to construe domestic legislation in such a way so as to accord with the interpretation which the European Court of Justice (ECJ) has given to any directive.

The extent to which the Equal Treatment Directive protects pregnant women was considered by the ECJ in *Dekker v Stichting Vormingscentrum Voor Junge Volwassenen*

(VJV – Centrum) Plus (1991) IRLR 27 ("Dekker") and *Handels og Kontorfunktionærenes Forbund i Danmark (acting for Hertz) v Dansk Arbejdsgiverforening (acting for Aldi Marked R/S)* 1991 IRLR 31 ("Hertz"). In both cases the ECJ indicated that any detrimental treatment on account of pregnancy would be in breach of the Equal Treatment Directive.

European Community Approach

In *Dekker*, the ECJ was faced with the case of Ms Dekker who, at her interview, openly informed her employers that she was pregnant. The interview panel nevertheless informed her that they would recommend her for the post since she was in their view the best candidate. However, when the review panel became aware of Ms Dekker's pregnancy, they decided not to employ her after all. The reason behind this was that the insurance policy which the employers had undertaken to cover maternity pay would not apply to Ms Dekker since she was pregnant before starting the job. The employers thought that they could not afford the financial consequences of engaging Ms Dekker. The ECJ held that the decision not to employ Ms Dekker constituted unlawful sex discrimination contrary to the Equal Treatment Directive.

> "As employment can only be refused because of pregnancy to a woman, such a refusal is direct discrimination on grounds of sex. A refusal to employ because of the financial consequences of absence connected with the pregnancy must be deemed to be based principally on the fact of the pregnancy."

The ECJ dismissed the argument that there could be no discrimination because pregnancy is a unique condition to women. Furthermore, it stated that it was of no significance that there were no male applicants since evidence of such discrimination is not contingent on comparing the treatment received by the woman with the treatment which a comparable man would have received. It was sufficient that the act of discrimination had occurred solely because Ms Dekker was pregnant and that if such a decision is taken, then that must be because she is a woman.

The ECJ also rejected the argument that the discrimination was not the employer's, but rather that of the terms of the insurance policy. The ECJ stated that no argument of financial burdens could excuse the employer's action.

Therefore, the ECJ unequivocally stated that it is direct contravention of Articles 2(1) and 3(1) of the Equal Treatment Directive 76/207 to refuse to appoint a woman because she is pregnant.

Equally, in *Hertz*, it was held that dismissal on grounds of pregnancy was direct discrimination. Mrs Hertz took her normal maternity leave entitlement and returned to work as scheduled. However, due to a number of complications caused by pregnancy and childbirth, she was repeatedly absent from work due to sickness arising from the pregnancy. As a result of these periods of absence, her employers dismissed her. The ECJ rejected her claim of sex discrimination on the grounds that the employer would have treated, and in fact had treated in the past, a man who had been absent due to sickness for a similar period of time, more favourably. They expressly rejected the argument that it was unlawful sex discrimination because the sickness absence was derived from her earlier difficult pregnancy and that male and female workers are equally exposed to illness and are treated equally in respect of time off work as a result.

In both *Dekker* and *Hertz*, the ECJ referred to a concept of a "protected period" for employees who are pregnant or on maternity leave. In *Hertz*, the ECJ stated that "it follows that during the maternity leave from which she benefits under national law, a woman is protected from dismissal because of her absence. It is a matter for each Member State to fix a period for maternity leave in such a way to allow female workers to be absent during the period during which problems due to pregnancy and confinement may arise".

The philosophy underlying the decision in *Dekker* and *Hertz* is that a woman should have the right not to be discriminated against on account of characteristics which are unique to the female sex. Therefore, an employer who treats a woman less favourably because of her pregnancy has committed an act of sex discrimination since the less favourable treatment flows from a condition which is unique to women. Therefore, pregnancy discrimination is automatically unlawful sex discrimination.

The English "Comparative" Approach

In *Webb v Emo Air Cargo (UK) Ltd (1993) IRLR 27*, the UK courts said that the correct test for determining whether adverse treatment because of pregnancy was on the grounds of sex and therefore amounted to unlawful sex discrimination was to ascertain whether the woman had been treated less favourably than a "comparable man" would have been treated in similar circumstances. The "comparable man" was to be a man of similar service who was sick or required hospital treatment involving a similar period of absence as the employee's maternity leave. If such a man would have retained his job in those circumstances, then so should the pregnant employee and a finding of unlawful sex discrimination would ensue. However, it is not unlawful sex discrimination if a man in the same relevant circumstances would have been treated similarly to the pregnant employee.

The respondent firm employed 16 employees with an import department of four employees. In June 1987, it became known that the import operations clerk, Mrs Stewart, was pregnant and would be taking up her statutory right to maternity leave at the end of the year. Consequently, Ms Webb was appointed as Mrs Stewart's replacement on 1 July. It was anticipated that Ms Webb would need approximately six months' training from Mrs Stewart prior to her taking her maternity leave. Her appointment was to be a permanent post since it was thought that she would remain in their employment after Mrs Stewart's return from maternity leave. However, several weeks after her appointment, Ms Webb discovered that she was also pregnant. She informed her employers of the situation and her employer formed the view that there was no other alternative available to them but to dismiss her. The firm did not deny that the dismissal was as a result of her pregnancy since the employer had written to her in the following terms: "Since you have only now told me that you are pregnant I have no alternative other than to terminate your employment with our company."

Ms Webb lodged a complaint to the industrial tribunal that she had been discriminated against on the grounds of sex. However, her complaint was dismissed by the industrial tribunal which held that the correct approach was to compare the treatment of Ms Webb with that which would have been accorded to a comparable man. It was held that if a man had been recruited instead of Ms Webb and had in similar circumstances informed his employers that he would have to be absent for a similar period of time, then that man would also have been dismissed. Therefore, the treatment accorded to Ms Webb was not on the grounds of her sex and she was not in fact treated less favourably than a man in similar circumstances would have been. The employers said that Ms Webb had been dismissed not simply because she was pregnant, but because she would need to be absent from work during the same period as Mrs Stewart whose position she had been recruited to fill in her absence.

The tribunal, on rejecting her claim that the company had acted contrary to the SDA, adopted the comparative approach laid down in the case of *Hayes*. The tribunal found that the real reason for Ms Webb's dismissal was that she would be absent from work at a crucial time and that although her pregnancy was the reason behind her absence from work, the employers would have treated a man with a similar need to be absent from work for such a period in exactly the same way.

Ms Webb appealed against this decision, however, the EAT dismissed the appeal, holding that if in similar circumstances a comparable man would have been treated in the same way as Ms Webb, then the treatment could not be on grounds of sex.

Ms Webb appealed to the Court of Appeal (CA), but this appeal was also dismissed. The CA held that the dismissal of a pregnant woman for a reason arising out of, or related to, the pregnancy could be, but is not necessarily, direct discrimination under s.1(1)(a). It was held that the industrial tribunal would have to find a man with "a condition as nearly comparable as possible which had the same practical effect upon his ability to do the job" and then to ask whether or not he would have been treated in the same way and dismissed.

However, between the decision of the EAT and the CA hearing in November 1992, the European Court of Justice (ECJ) had interpreted the meaning of the Equal Treatment Directive 76/207 in the cases of *Dekker* and *Hertz*. The conclusion was that the Directive does not require a "comparable man" since pregnancy is unique to women and so any less favourable treatment on this basis is direct discrimination. Despite this decision, the CA in *Webb* nevertheless maintained that they could adopt their interpretation of the SDA and the need for a "comparable man" without conflicting with the decision of the ECJ.

The case then went to the House of Lords due to the arguments which had arisen as to the potential inconsistency between the domestic law, established in *Webb* and the law in *Dekker* and *Hertz*.

The House of Lords adopted a very different approach than that adopted by the EAT and the CA. The House of Lords did not endorse the comparative approach, in fact, to the contrary. Lord Keith's decision for their Lordships stated that:

> *"There can be no doubt that in general to dismiss a woman because she is pregnant or to refuse to employ a woman of child-bearing age because she may become pregnant is unlawful direct discrimination. Child-bearing and the capacity for child-bearing are characteristic of the female sex. So to apply these characteristics as the criterion for dismissal or refusal to employ is to apply a gender-based criterion which the majority of this House in James v Eastleigh Borough Council (1990) IRLR 288 held to constitute unlawful direct discrimination."*

However, Lord Keith went on to say that in Ms Webb's case "there was not any direct application of a gender-based criterion." This was because she was dismissed not simply since she was pregnant, but because of the fact that as a result of her pregnancy she would not be available to work during the period for which her cover was needed. It was held that in such circumstances the comparable man is required in order to assess how he would have been treated in the same situation. Therefore, the distinction which the House of Lords seems to be making is that where a dismissal occurs on grounds of pregnancy that is automatically unlawful discrimination without the necessity for the comparable man. However, where the dismissal is as a result of the consequences of the pregnancy then the comparable man approach should be adopted to establish how he would have been treated.

It appears, therefore, that the House of Lords is saying that a comparable man is only necessary when the employer is acting on a gender-neutral factor. The House of Lords on 26 November 1992 adjourned the appeal and referred the following question to the ECJ for a preliminary ruling.

> *"Is it discrimination on grounds of sex contrary to Directive 76/207 for an employer to dismiss a female employee (the appellant):*
>
> (a) *whom he engaged for the specific purpose of replacing (after training) another female employee during the latter's forthcoming maternity leave*
>
> (b) *when very shortly after the appointment, the employer discovers that the appellant herself will be absent on maternity leave during the maternity leave of the other employee, and the employer dismisses her because he needs the job-holder to be at work during that period*
>
> (c) *had the employer known of the pregnancy of the appellant at the date of the appointment, she would not have been appointed, and*
>
> (d) *the employer would similarly have dismissed a male employee engaged for this purpose who required leave of absence at the relevant time for medical or other reasons?"*

Many commentators argue that the decision in *Webb* is contrary to and at odds with the decisions in *Dekker* and *Hertz*. Realistically, very few dismissals of pregnant employees occur simply because the employee is pregnant.

In reality, the dismissals occur in response to the actual consequences of the pregnancy, such as maternity leave and the payment of SMP.

The Advocate General, whose opinion is often followed by the European Court, indicated that the questions posed by the House of Lords in the *Webb* case should be answered in the affirmative, namely that there would be a breach of the Equal Treatment Directive if an employee is dismissed for any reason related to pregnancy and that this would cover the facts of the *Webb* case itself. However, in his opinion, the Advocate General did not appear to address the issue of whether such an interpretation would cover both private as well as public sector employees.

As anticipated, the European Court of Justice (ECJ) ruled that the dismissal of a pregnant woman employed under what the ECJ calls an "indefinite contract" is in breach of the Equal Treatment Directive and that it is wrong to compare the position of a pregnant woman to that of a comparable man.

Questions and Answers

Q: In England what approach is adopted by the courts in the past in assessing whether a pregnant employee has been a victim of sex discrimination?

A: *The "comparative" approach. A pregnant employee is compared to a man who has a medical condition requiring him to be absent from work for a similar period of time as the pregnant employee. If the woman has been treated less favourably than the "comparable man" a finding of unlawful sex discrimination would be made. If the "comparable man" had been treated in the same way as the pregnant employee then the treatment cannot be discriminatory on grounds of sex.*

Q: To what extent should UK law be interpreted in a manner consistent with European Law?

A: *Case law has stated that UK courts and tribunals are obliged to construe domestic legislation in accordance with EC Directives. However, that is on the proviso that it is possible to do so without distorting the meaning of the UK legislation.*

Q: How did the ECJ interpret the Equal Treatment Directive in the cases* Dekker *and* Hertz?

A: *The Directive does not require a "comparable man". The ECJ said that pregnancy is unique to women and any less favourable treatment of a pregnant employee because of the pregnancy is undoubtedly direct sex discrimination.*

Q: What the House of Lords say about the potential inconsistency between domestic law in *Webb* and EEC law in *Dekker* and *Hertz*?

A: *The House of Lords stated that where the dismissal of a pregnant employee is on grounds of pregnancy, this is* *automatically unlawful discrimination and there is no need for a "comparable man". However, where the dismissal is as a result of the pregnancy, a "comparative man" approach should be adopted in order to establish how a "comparable man" would have been treated.*

Q: What is the current position?

A: *The ECJ ruling has confirmed that the "comparable man" approach is discriminatory. That it is a breach of the Equal Treatment Directive to dismiss a woman because she is pregnant or will be temporarily unavailable for work for that reason.*

3 Maternity Leave and the Right to Return to Work

Introduction

Prior to the Trade Union Reform and Employment Rights Act 1993 (TURERA 1993), there was no statutory right in UK law to maternity leave for an employee who has less than two years service. It has been argued, however, that such a right might exist under the Equal Treatment Directive. Support for this view might exist under the European Court of Justice's (ECJ) decision in *Dekker* (see page 23). In that case, the employers refused to appoint a pregnant employee because of the financial consequences which would have flowed from her appointment. The ECJ considered that, nonetheless, the reason for her non-appointment related to her sex and appeared to hold that a refusal to appoint on grounds of pregnancy amounted to a breach of the Equal Treatment Directive. By analogy, the same argument could be applied to a woman who wanted to take or return from maternity leave.

The ECJ's approach contrasts to the approach taken up to now by UK courts to claims under sex discrimination law. The UK courts in the past have taken the view that conduct will only be discriminatory if it can be shown that a man would have been treated more favourably in comparable circumstances. For example in *Webb v EMO Air Cargo (UK) Ltd (1993) IRLR 27* (see page 25) the House of Lords ruled that the industrial tribunal was entitled to find that Ms Webb had not been discriminated against on the basis that a man who had been employed to provide temporary cover for an employee during a period of authorised absence would also have been dismissed if he had requested time off for an operation. In other words, Ms Webb had not been dismissed because of her pregnancy, but because she was not available for work and that a man would have been dismissed in comparable circumstances. The House of Lords, however, referred the matter to the ECJ, and as anticipated the ECJ ruled that the dismissal of a pregnant woman employed under an "indefinite contract" is in breach of the Equal Treatment Directive and that it is wrong to compare the position of a pregnant woman to a comparable man. It remains to be seen how the ECJ's judgement will be interpreted and applied in practice and in particular whether it will mean that women will be entitled to receive all their rights including contractual pay and benefits during a period of maternity leave.

The New Right to Short-term Maternity Leave

As a result of the EC Pregnant Workers Directive, the Government has been forced to change UK law to give all employees a right to a 14 week minimum period of maternity leave irrespective of their length of service. The new law affects women whose expected week of confinement (EWC) falls on or after 16 October 1994.

Those employees who have two or more years' continuous employment at the 11th week before the EWC will continue to be entitled to long-term maternity leave for a period up to a maximum of 40 weeks. The provisions relating to long-term maternity leave are considered on page 43. Although the notification and other conditions attached to short-term and long-term maternity leave are similar, there are some differences and there are important differences in the concept underlying the two types of maternity leave.

The new provisions for short-term maternity leave appear to be drafted on the assumption that such leave is a form of "authorised absence" and therefore the contract of employment continues to regulate the employment relationship in the pregnant employee's absence in much the same way as it would do if the pregnant employee was on sick leave or some other form of authorised absence. The statutory provisions make it clear that all the terms of employment, except for payment of salary (and possibly some other forms of remuneration), will continue to apply during the period of absence.

However, in the case of long-term maternity leave, the statutory scheme assumes that the employment relationship would have ended but for the protection given by the provisions themselves. The provisions therefore assume that the contract itself either comes to an end or is suspended during the period of maternity leave, and the statutory provision in effect provides for the reinstatement of the employee at the end of her period of maternity leave. This has a number of important practical implications in relation to any "entitlement" to benefits during the maternity leave period.

Despite the new statutory rights, the issues raised in the *Webb* case will continue to be relevant in four situations.

- Whether it is lawful not to recruit someone who is pregnant not for reasons of pregnancy as such but because of her unavailability for work.

- Employees who do not qualify for long-term maternity leave but are off work for maternity related reasons for more than 14 weeks.

- The benefits received by employees during a period of long-term maternity leave.

- Employees who seek to come back after a period of long-term maternity leave and who threaten sex discrimination proceedings if their employers refuse to take them back.

The Right to Short-term Maternity Leave

As stated above, a woman whose EWC is 16 October 1994 or after, irrespective of her length of service will have the right to a minimum 14 week maternity leave period.

When does the Right Accrue?

TURERA 1993 refers to "an employee". Until an individual has actually started work she cannot be regarded as an employee even if she has received a job offer. As soon, however, as the contract of employment has commenced then she is an employee. An employer would, therefore, be obliged to give maternity leave to a member of staff who announced herself pregnant on the first day of her employment!

The Statutory Maternity Leave Period

The statutory maternity leave period starts on the date chosen by the prospective mother and notified to her employer provided that the date is not earlier than the 11th week before the EWC and not later than the day on which the baby is born.

However, the Government was concerned that by leaving the choice of notified date in the hands of the prospective mother, it would be possible for a woman who suffers a pregnancy-related illness to postpone the start of her 14 week maternity leave period and claim sick pay until the baby is born. To prevent this, the Act provides that any absence for a pregnancy-related reason after the sixth week before the EWC will trigger the statutory maternity leave period. To ensure that the employer is aware of the reason for the pregnant women's absence, the statute requires a woman who is off work due to pregnancy or childbirth after the beginning of the sixth week before the EWC to notify her employer as soon as is reasonably practicable that she was absent for that reason.

The provisions do appear, however, to have the strange result that if an employee is off work for one day for a pregnancy-related reason after the six week deadline, the maternity leave period is automatically triggered with the result that the employee has no right to return to work in the period before the baby is born (even if she wants to) unless the employers agree to allow her to return.

These rules only take effect from the beginning of the sixth week before the EWC, so a woman who is sick for a pregnancy-related illness may continue to receive sick pay until that time without her statutory maternity leave being triggered.

Requirement to Inform Employer of Pregnancy

A prospective mother does not have the right to short-term maternity leave unless she informs her employer in writing at least 21 days before her maternity leave period begins that:

- she is pregnant
- the EWC (or if the baby has been born, the date of birth), and
- if the employer so requests, produces a certificate from a registered medical practitioner or registered midwife stating the expected week of childbirth.

Sometimes it is not possible to comply with these provisions, for example if the baby is born prematurely. In such circumstances, the employee is under a duty to notify the employer as soon as is "reasonably practicable".

A failure to comply with these provisions will mean that the employee will cease to be protected by the legislation once she has left work and will have no statutory right to return.

Notification of Commencement of Maternity Leave

A prospective mother is also required, at least 21 days before the commencement of her maternity leave (or if this is not reasonably practicable, as soon as is reasonably practicable), to notify her employer of the date on which she wishes her maternity leave to start.

However, as the provisions make clear, this date cannot be earlier than 11 weeks before the EWC unless the baby is premature, in which case the notice may be given "as soon as is reasonably practicable after the birth".

As noted above, the maternity leave period may be triggered off at an earlier date if the female employee is off work for a reason related to pregnancy or childbirth after the sixth week before the EWC.

In contrast to the requirement to inform the employer of pregnancy, this notification need not be in writing unless the employer so requests.

A failure to comply with these provisions will mean that the employee will cease to be protected by the statutory provisions once she has left work.

Reasonably practicable

Both the requirement to inform and the requirement to notify are subject to the qualification that it is "reasonably practicable" to do so. It has been established in unfair dismissal cases that this is a comparatively strict test and there is no discretion in the tribunal to waive the notification requirement where it would be just and equitable to do so. However, it would cover situations where it is not practicable to notify the employer where the employee is hospitalised or physically prevented from notifying the employer for some reason and tribunals are likely to be fairly sympathetic to the individual where the failure to notify is related to pregnancy and childbirth.

Absence Prior to the Eleventh Week Before Expected Week of Childbirth

The Act is silent as to how such an absence is to be treated, so the assumption is that such an absence should be treated as sickness absence under the employer's standard sickness procedure.

Length of Maternity Leave

The maternity leave period (MLP) will last for 14 weeks from the commencement date, or until the birth of the child, whichever is the later.

However, in the following circumstances the MLP may be longer than 14 weeks where:

- there is a contractual entitlement to a longer maternity leave period

- the employee qualifies for long-term maternity leave in accordance with the statutory provisions (see page 43)

- the baby is overdue, in which case the MLP is extended to the date of birth plus a minimum period of two weeks. It is unlawful for a woman to return to work less than two weeks after childbirth. This period is increased to four weeks where a woman works in a factory

- a mother is prohibited from returning to work for health and safety reasons related to having recently given birth. In such circumstances, the maternity leave period will continue until it is safe for her return

- the woman is unable to return for medical reasons (see below).

Extension for Medical Reasons

An employer may not dismiss an employee within four weeks of the 14 weeks return date where the reason for dismissal is that the employee has given birth to a child, or any other reason connected with her having given birth to a child (for example, postnatal depression) if:

- she has, before the end of her MLP, provided a medical certificate stating that she would be incapable of work after the end of that period, and

- she remains incapable of work and the medical certificate remains current (s.24 TURERA).

It should be noted, however, that these provisions protect a woman from being dismissed during the four week period but do not entitle her to receive contractual benefits during the extended period.

Other Grounds

It should not be assumed that it is automatically fair to dismiss someone who fails to return at the end of the maternity leave period as there may be other explanations for her failure to return which might lead to claims for unfair dismissal or allegations of sex discrimination. This is particularly important in relation to women who qualify for protection against unfair dismissal during the maternity leave period, ie those who did not have two years service before they went on maternity leave but qualify during their MLP.

A woman might be able to bring a sex discrimination claim if the reason for her failure to return is unrelated to her maternity leave as would be the case if she was involved in a car accident or had her home broken into and could show that a man would have been allowed additional time off work in comparable circumstances. She might even be able to argue that a man who underwent an operation would have been given additional time off in comparable circumstances, or on a liberal interpretation of *Webb* that she was still protected against dismissal during her extended period of maternity leave under the Equal Treatment Directive.

Early Return

An employee who intends to return to work earlier than the end of her maternity leave period is required to give her employer at least seven days notice of the date on which she intends to return. Failure to do so entitles her employer to postpone her return until the seven day period has expired although this must not go beyond the end of the maternity leave period. If the employee attempts to return early, having been told not to do so by her employer, the employer is under "no contractual obligation to pay her remuneration until the date on which she may return".

Contractual Rights During Maternity

During the MLP, an employee is "entitled to the benefit of the terms and conditions of employment which would have been applicable to her if she had not been absent" excluding "any entitlement to remuneration".

This means that women on short-term maternity leave are entitled to receive all their contractual benefits, ie to be treated as if they were still at work. This is consistent with the idea that short-term maternity leave is a form of authorised absence. So, for example, a sales representative who was entitled to a company car would be entitled to keep her company car during her MLP. Similarly, a woman would continue to accrue holiday during her MLP, or any other service-related benefit.

However, the right to "remuneration" during the MLP is excluded. The idea behind the exclusion was to ensure that the statutory provisions dovetail with the new rules on SMP (see page 83) but there is some uncertainty as to what is meant by "remuneration" in this context.

The intention was to make it quite clear that remuneration was limited to wages and salaries, rather than other forms of payment or benefits which an employee receives. However, in the context of schedule 14 to the Employment Protection (Consolidation) Act 1978 (EP(C)A), remuneration has been held to cover commission, bonuses, profit shares and other payments received by the employee under her contract of employment. It remains to be seen whether tribunals follow this approach. The Government has, however, stated that occupational pensions are not "remuneration" and that therefore pension contributions remain payable during the maternity leave period. A woman must continue to accrue benefits under the pension scheme as if she were working normally. If she contributes to the scheme her contributions may be based on her actual rate of pay including statutory maternity pay.

SMP Entitlement

Since the 14 week MLP is shorter than the 18 week period of entitlement to SMP, if the employee returns to work after the 14 week period she would be entitled to her contracted pay and so the 4 weeks remaining SMP would not be effective.

Right to Return

Unlike long-term maternity leave (see page 43), there is no statutory right to return to the same job on the same terms and conditions as such, but the same result is achieved because it is automatically unfair to dismiss a woman if her "maternity leave period is ended by [her] dismissal and the reason for her dismissal is that she has given birth to a child or any other reason connected with her having given birth to a child". So, if the employer refuses to allow the woman to return to work at the end of the maternity leave period, she will be treated as having been unfairly dismissed. Furthermore, in contrast with long-term maternity leave, there is no requirement for the employee to notify her employer of her return at the end of her MLP. The period of leave is fixed and so her return date (if she returns) is certain.

Similarly, although there is no statutory right to return on the same terms and conditions, a woman who is not allowed to return to the same job on the same terms and conditions could claim that she had been constructively dismissed and her constructive dismissal would be unfair if the reason for the employers action was in any way connected with childbirth.

The provisions do not, however, prevent an employer from going ahead with changes in terms and conditions which are unconnected with the childbirth as might be the case where there is reorganisation of the business in the employee's absence. Similarly, there is no right to return when the position is redundant, although an individual has the right to be offered suitable alternative employment in such circumstances (see page 59).

Contractual Right to Maternity Leave

There is nothing to prevent an employer from offering more generous maternity leave terms than those laid down by the statutory provisions. For example, some employers offer more generous maternity pay than the minimum laid down in the statutory provisions. In such circumstances, the employee is able to choose whichever of the two rights is the more favourable to her.

Checklist: Short-term Maternity Leave

- The right accrues from day 1 of employment.
- The employee must notify the employer 21 days before leave is due to start or as soon as practicable.
- It is for an obligatory 14 weeks unless the employee gives at least seven days' written notice of a return before the 14th week.
- It cannot start earlier than the 11th week before the EWC or upon the actual birth.
- The employer can postpone an early return by seven days.
- If a sicknote has been presented before the 14 week period expires and it remains in force, the MLP can last for an additional four weeks.
- The employer must pay SMP.
- The employee is entitled to the benefit of all the terms of her contract except pay during this period.
- The employee is entitled to any contractual benefits over and above the statutory framework which her contract may provide.

Long-term Maternity Leave

In addition to the new right to short-term maternity leave, those who have two or more years' continuous employment at the 11th week before the EWC are entitled to a further period of 26 weeks maternity leave making a total of 40 weeks in all. Subject to certain conditions, s.39 of the EP(C)A (now substituted by TURERA, s.23 sch.2) gives a woman the right to return to work at the end of the period of maternity leave on terms which are no less favourable than those which she enjoyed before she left. Similarly, her continuity of employment is preserved during the period of maternity leave, but the position regarding her contract and in particular any continuing rights she has to benefit during the period of long-term maternity leave is less clear cut (see page 47).

The Right to Long-term Maternity Leave

A woman qualifies for long-term maternity leave (and the right to return to work thereafter) if she satisfies the following conditions:

- she continues to be employed by her employer (whether or not she is at work) until immediately before the 11th week before the EWC

- she has at the beginning of the 11th week before the EWC been employed either for a period of at least 2 years provided she works 16 hours or more, or for a period of 5 years or more provided she works between 8 hours and 16 hours

- she complies with the notification requirements referred to below.

Continuously Employed until Immediately before the 11th Week

The condition that an employee must "continue to be employed until immediately before the 11th week before the EWC" is satisfied regardless of whether the employee is actually at work. There may be a number of reasons as to why an employee is not actually at work immediately before the beginning of the 11th week, for example she may be on holiday or on sick leave. Nevertheless, her contract of employment continues to exist and she remains employed even though she is not physically present at work.

Notification Requirements

The right to long-term maternity leave is conditional on the individual complying with the various statutory notification requirements which arise both before she takes maternity leave and during maternity leave. Failure to comply with one or more of these notification requirements will mean that the employee loses the right to return and ceases to be protected under the legislation.

- **Requirement to inform employer of pregnancy**

The employee must inform the employer in writing at least 21 days before her maternity leave period begins (or if that is not practicable, as soon as is reasonably practicable) that she is pregnant, the EWC (or if the baby has already been born, the date on which the baby was born) *and that she intends to return to work*. If the employer so requires, she may be required to produce a medical certificate from a registered medical practitioner or a registered midwife stating the EWC. These requirements are the same as those in relation to short-term maternity leave, except that the employee is required to make it clear that she intends to exercise the right to return.

- **Notification of commencement of maternity leave**

These requirements are the same as those in relation to short-term maternity leave, except that the employee is required also to make it clear that she intends to exercise the right to return.

- **Notification during maternity leave**

A woman on long-term maternity leave may be asked to confirm that she intends to return to work. The request from her employer must be in writing and must include a warning about the consequences of failing to reply, ie that the right to return will be lost. It cannot be made earlier than 21 days before the end of the 14 week MLP and the employee must reply in writing within 14 days of receiving the request (or as soon as is reasonably practicable thereafter). It should be noted that whilst confirmation of return cannot be requested earlier than 21 days before the end of the MLP, the timing of childbirth together with the commencement of the MLP may make this impractical. For example, a woman who commenced her MLP period 11 weeks before the EWC could be asked for a written confirmation of her intention to return at the approximate time of childbirth. In these circumstances employers would receive a more realistic assessment of the employee's intentions by making such a request further into the extended maternity leave period.

- **Employees failure to comply with notification requirements**

The tribunals have taken a strict approach to compliance with these notification requirements. For example, in *FW Woolworth plc v Smith (1990) ICR 45* the EAT found that since the employee had failed to state an actual intention to return to work and had simply provided the employer with a "certificate of expected confinement", she had not satisfied the notice requirements and had lost her statutory right to return.

A harsh approach was taken in the case of *Osbourne v Thomas Bolton & Sons Ltd COIT 794/248* where the employee was diabetic who had been warned that there was a chance that the pregnancy could have complications. As a result of this potential complication she simply informed her employer that if she lost the child she would return to work. This notification did not satisfy the tribunal who stated that a conditional notice is inadequate.

It is, therefore, advisable for an employee to protect her position and keep her option open by indicating that she intends to return to work, since she can of course change her mind at a later date.

Late Notification

Late notification will not automatically mean that an employee has lost her right to return to work so long as she can show that it was not "reasonably practicable" for her to comply with the time period and that she gave notice as soon as she possibly could in the circumstances. It is evident that tribunals have a tendency to take a rather strict view as regards the employees compliance with these time limits although exception is made in certain instances, for example where the employee has had to leave work prematurely due to complications with her pregnancy.

Timing of Absence

An employee is entitled to commence her maternity leave at any time after the 11th week before the EWC.

There is no restriction on an employee working beyond the 11th week and thereby delaying her maternity leave. An employee can insist on delaying her maternity leave and her employer does not have the right to insist that she leave at the 11th week. This is the case even where there is a contractual provision to the contrary since any such contractual requirement on the employee to leave employment after the 11th week would contravene s.140 of the EP(C)A. However, if absence after the 6th week is due to the pregnancy or a pregnancy-related reason then maternity leave can be deemed to have started.

Status of the Contract during Maternity Leave

The statutory scheme leaves open the question whether the contract of employment continues whilst a women is on long-term maternity leave. This will be determined by her actions and those of her employer and in particular by what has been expressly or impliedly agreed between the parties.

Where, for example, the employee has resigned or has been dismissed before or during her maternity leave, it is clear that the contract of employment will come to an end. However, it should be noted that where an employee resigns after the 11th week before her EWC, she still has the right to treat her absence as due to pregnancy and will therefore still qualify for long-term maternity leave. Similarly, if the woman is dismissed before or during her maternity leave, she is still entitled to statutory protection.

On the other hand where the parties expressly or impliedly agreed to continue to observe the terms of the contract in the employee's absence, the contract will remain in force during the maternity leave. For example, in *Ryan v Sporting Tours Promotions Ltd (unreported)*, the employee was paid 10 weeks' sick pay whilst she was on maternity leave. The tribunal held that the contract had not come to an end when the maternity leave had begun, but continued to subsist during the period of maternity leave. Similarly, an agreement may be reached which allows the employee to retain the company car during her maternity leave and to continue to receive other benefits under her contract. In such circumstances the contract will continue to be in existence. Furthermore, the continued existence of the contract may be tacitly acknowledged by, for example putting the employee on the pay roll. The balance of authority therefore appears to favour the view that, unless the employee resigns or is dismissed, or her status during maternity leave is expressly agreed between the parties, the contract of employment will be suspended during the period of maternity leave *(Institute of the Motor Industry v Harvey [1992] IRLR 343).*

This has the following consequences.

- There is no right to receive any payments or benefits under the contract. For example, there is no contractual right to retain the company car beyond the period of short-term maternity leave. However, to avoid sex discrimination claims, employers must ensure that their treatment of female employees on maternity leave is consistent with their treatment of male employees on sick leave. A claim for sex discrimination succeeded in *Reay v Sunderland Health Authority (unreported)* where an industrial tribunal held that a woman health visitor returning to work from maternity leave was entitled to time off in lieu for bank holidays which fell during her maternity absence because her male comparators were entitled to time off in lieu for bank holidays which fell during their sick leave.
- The employee can complain of constructive dismissal if the employer acts in a manner which undermines the mutual trust and confidence between the parties.
- The employee can complain of unfair dismissal even though she may have lost her statutory right to return *(Hilton International Hotels UK Ltd v Kaissi 1994) IRLR 270.*

Confirmation of Intention to Return

The employee's requirement to confirm with the employer her intention to return to work is strict and if an employee fails to comply with or follow the specified time limit she will lose her right to return unless she can show that it was not reasonably practicable for her to comply.

The request to the employee must be in writing and warn of the implication of her failure to respond, namely that she will automatically lose her right to return to work unless she provides written confirmation to her employer within the 14 days of the employer requesting such confirmation. However, there is the proviso that if that is not reasonably practicable, then as soon as is reasonably practicable thereafter.

Checklist: Confirmation of Intention to Return

Letter to employee seeking confirmation of intention to return should:

- Ask her to confirm intention to return.

- Inform her that should she not comply with this request within 14 days, she will forfeit her right to return.

- Enclose S.A.E. (optional).

Letter not to be sent earlier than 21 days before the end of the basic leave period. See Figure 3 for model letter.

Notification of Date of Return

The time-scale for giving notification of the date of return is much stricter than as regards the first notification and the confirmation of return discussed above. The employee can not rely on the escape clause that it was not reasonably practicable to so to comply with the time limit. Therefore, failure to comply results in her forfeiting her statutory right to return. Notification to the employer **must** be given in writing at least 21 days before the day on which she intends to return. The date is referred to as the "notified day of return" (NDR) and must be stated in the notice. Care needs to be taken by the employee — the NDR must be before the last day of the 29th week beginning with the week the EWC fell. There is no escape clause so that if an employee fails to comply with the time limit she will automatically lose her right to return to work.

Postponement of Date of Return

In limited circumstances, both the employer and employee have a right to postpone the employee's return to work beyond the 29th week.

Postponement by Employee

An employee may postpone her return if:

> "she gives the employer a certificate from a registered medical practitioner stating that by reasons of disease or bodily or mental disablement she will be incapable of work on the notified day of return or the expiration of that period, as the case may be". — Schedule 2, Section 42(3) TURERA 1993

A postponement under this section may be for up to four weeks from the NDR or, if she has not provided an NDR, then her postponement can extend no further than four weeks from the expiration of the original 29 weeks of maternity leave.

The employee is required to produce a medical certificate either before the NDR or before the end of the 29 weeks if she had not provided an NDR. The production of a medical certificate is mandatory and there is no escape clause for the employee, even if it is not reasonably practicable for her to produce one. Therefore, even if the medical certificate is dated only one day after the end of the 29 week period, this is nevertheless a breach of the statutory requirements and consequently the employee would lose her right to return.

An employee can only take advantage of this postponement ONCE. An employee who has so exercised her right is not be entitled to again postpone or extend the date of her return to work. This statutory provision creates a number of problems and an employer can regard an employee as having exercised her right of postponement even if the postponement has not been for a period of four weeks. For example, an employee who requests a postponement for only one week will be treated as having exercised her right despite the postponement being for one week only and she is not entitled to postpone for a further three weeks at a later date in order to take up her full entitlement to four weeks. Once one postponement has been exercised, regardless of the length of time of that postponement, that is the end of the matter and the right has been exhausted.

However, there is an exception where the statutory right to the four weeks postponement can be extended by agreement between the parties. For example, in *Dowuona v John Lewis Plc 1987 ICR 788*, the employee was contractually entitled to an additional week's holiday leave on top of her statutory right for four week's postponement of return to work. She exercised her right to postpone her return for four weeks and she added on her additional one week holiday entitlement under her contract. However, at the end of that five weeks, the employee was still not well enough to return to work and so on her return at a later date it was held by the Court of Appeal that she had in fact lost her right to return since it was maternity leave from which she was returning and not holiday leave.

An exception will also occur if the contract of employment expressly permits more than one postponement.

The Northern Ireland Equal Opportunities Commission are currently supporting cases which contend that the statutory framework of the return to work regulations are contrary to the provisions of the Equal Treatment Directive. They assert that a refusal to allow a return to work after the 29 week period (or 4 week sickness extension) is sex discrimination. It remains to be seen whether this view will be accepted in the light of the *Webb* decision.

Period of Interruption

Schedule 2, s. 42(5) TURERA 1993 states that:

> "If an employee has notified a date of return but there is an interruption of work (whether due to industrial action or some other reason) which renders it unreasonable to expect the employee to return to work on the notified day of return, she may instead return to work when work resumes after the interruption or as soon as reasonably practicable afterwards."

"Interruption of work" is not specifically defined in the Act other than that it may be as a result of "industrial action or some other reason".

There is no limitation on the number of occasions that postponement can be exercised on this ground.

Neither the employer nor the employee is required to nominate a new return date since the return under this provision is postponed automatically until either the interruption ends or until as soon as it is "reasonably practicable" to return. The reasons for it not being reasonably practicable for the employee to return to work should be connected with the operation of the business and not for any other reason connected to the personal circumstances of the employee. As discussed earlier, if an employee is too unwell to return to work she can request a postponement.

If no NDR has been submitted by the employee and it seems likely that the interruption will prevent her from returning to work after the expiration of the 29 weeks period, she is entitled to exercise her right so that she returns to work at any time before the end of a period of 28 days from the date of the interruption and it is of no effect that she is actually returning to work outside the 29 week period.

Postponement by Employer

Schedule 2, s.42(2) TURERA 1993 states:

> "An employer may postpone an employee's return to work until a date not more than four weeks after the notified day of return. If he notifies her before that day that for specified reasons he is postponing her return until that date, and accordingly she will be entitled to return to work with him on that date."

The employee must be notified of this postponement before the NDR and she must be told the reasons for the postponement and the day upon which she may return to work.

There is no requirement for the employer to notify the employee in writing. "Specified reasons" have been held not to be limited to matters arising or connected with the employee's maternity leave, but could include the employer's general business requirements.

An employee may find an employer postponing her return by more than the statutory four weeks. In practice, employers are not legally entitled to do this and it will amount to a "deemed" dismissal if an employee, having exercised her right to return to work, is not permitted to do so. However, if an employee has entered into agreement with the employer for an extension of this four week period then she has *not* been dismissed. In addition, any claim an employee may make for loss of earnings in the period beyond the statutory four weeks should be proceeded in the County Court.

It is possible for the three postponement situations described above to occur in relation to the same period of the employee's maternity leave. If this is the case, then the NDR is to be taken as being the last day in which her return is postponed.

The Right to Return to What?

Section 39(2) as substituted by s.23 and Sch. 2 TURERA 1993 states that where an employee has been absent from work, either wholly or partly because of pregnancy or confinement, her right to return to work is subject to a number of provisions contained in that section. Broadly speaking, it is the right to return to work to do the job she was doing before, at the salary she would have been getting (and indeed with all other terms and benefits) had she not been absent at all but had carried on working during that period.

Section 39(2) as substituted by s.23 and Sch. 2 TURERA 1993 states:

> "A right to return to work under this section is the right to return to work with that person who was her employer before the end of her maternity leave period, or (where appropriate) his successor, in the job which she was employed:
>
> (a) on terms and conditions not less favourable than those which would have been applicable to her if she had not been absent from work at any time since the commencement of her maternity leave period
>
> (b) with her seniority, pension rights and similar rights as they would have been if the period or periods of her employment prior to the end of her maternity leave period were continuous with her employment following her return to work (but subject to the requirements of paragraph 5 of Schedule 5 to the Society Security Act 1989 (credit for the period of absence in certain cases)), and
>
> (c) otherwise on terms and conditions no less favourable than those which would have been applicable to her had she not been absent from work after the end of her maternity leave period."

There is no question of reasonableness on behalf of the employer or consideration of what is economical for the employer — failure to permit an employee to return is automatically unfair dismissal.

An employee returning to work is entitled to treat the period of employment prior to the employee's absence for the purposes of retaining her seniority, pension rights and other similar rights. Therefore, each week whilst the employee is on maternity leave shall count towards computing her continuity of employment. An employee, therefore, must benefit from any pay increase which fellow colleagues have been granted during her absence and at the same time she will also be subject to any decrease or general deterioration of contractual terms which would have equally affected her had she not been on maternity leave.

An employee may also have contractual rights as regards her return to work as well as the rights contained in the EP(C)A. However, she may not "exercise the two rights separately but may in returning to work take advantage of whatever right is, in any particular respect, the more favourable" — Section 44(1), as substituted by s.23 (1)(b), Sch. 2 TURERA 1993.

Same Job

The word "job" is defined in s.153(1) EP(C)A 1978 and refers to it as being "the nature of the work which he (the employee) is employed to do in accordance with his contract and the capacity and place in which he is so employed".

It has been successfully argued that, as a result of the definition of the word "job" referred to above, an employee returning from maternity leave does not have the right to return to exactly the same job as she was doing before she left and that an employer could move an employee to work for someone else so long as it was the same type of work, at the same place of work and at the same level within the company.

Minor changes in job description are likely to be ignored. For example, in *Edgell v Lloyds Register of Shipping [1977] IRLR 463*, Ms Edgell was a bookkeeper who before her maternity leave, had reported directly to her departmental manager. On her return she found that, as a result of a reorganisation, she no longer had authority to sign cheques and had to report to a supervisor. The industrial tribunal, however, considered that the changes in her job were insufficient to amount to a change in the nature of her work.

However, the statutory provisions will be infringed if an employer takes an employee back after her maternity leave on inferior terms. For example, in *Castles Walker v Northern Cooperation Society Ltd (unreported)*, a tribunal found that the job of confidential secretary to the chief accountant, which Ms Castles was offered on her return from maternity leave, was not the same as her original post of confidential secretary to the chief executive officer because it involved a reduction in status.

An employer who takes an employee back after her maternity leave on inferior terms is infringing the employee's rights under this statutory provision.

At the same time, there are also obligations on the employee on her return to carry out her contract as before and so she has no right to return to work and request reduced or varied hours on the basis that she now has new responsibilities at home which require this. Although, an employee may have a claim under the Sex Discrimination Act 1975 for indirect sex discrimination under such circumstances if such an application is not properly considered, *Holmes v Home Office 1984, IRLR 299*.

Nature of Work

The exact definition of "nature of work" obviously depends to a large extent on what is stated in the contract. It follows, therefore, that if there is a job flexibility clause entitling the employer to move employees to a different type of work, or to vary their responsibilities, then an employer is perfectly entitled to offer that different work to an employee on her return from maternity leave. For example, in *Llewellyn v Wigglesworth Ltd (unreported)*, a tribunal decided that Ms Llewellyn had not been permitted to return to her old job as a sales representative when the job she was given covered a wider area.

Place of Work

An employee's place of work depends on the terms of the contract and whether the employer has a right to move the employee to a different place of work in accordance with the terms of the contract. If there is no such right, then the employee will have a right to return to the job she was doing at her old place of work.

Duty to Reinstate

A refusal by an employer to either give an employee returning from her maternity leave the "same" job as she had been employed in prior to her absence, or not permitting her to return to work at all, is automatically a dismissal, subject to the proviso that the employee has complied with all the statutory notice provisions outlined earlier. She is treated as having been dismissed with effect from her NDR. Section 56 is relevant where the employee is bringing an unfair dismissal claim under Part V of the Act. Section 86 is where the employee is making a claim for a redundancy payment under Part VI of the Act.

Failure to Permit Return Amounts to Dismissal

Section 56 of the EP(C)A provides that where an employee is entitled to return to work in accordance with the statutory provision, but is not permitted to return, she will be treated as having been employed until her notified day of return and as dismissed from that day for the reason for which she was not permitted to return.

However, in two situations the employee is treated by the statutory provisions as not having been dismissed and therefore is unable to bring a claim.

Small Employers

There is an exception to s.56 in the case of employers with five or less employees (including employees of any associated employer).

This exception arose as a result of protests by small employers about the maternity legislation and the right of an employee to complain of unfair dismissal in respect of her return to work after maternity leave. They claimed that it was difficult and expensive for them to administer. Unlike larger firms they did not have the resources to train a temporary replacement and then have to reinstate an employee after her maternity leave. Because a small company does not have the personnel to be able to allocate the work of an employee taking maternity leave among the other employees it is generally necessary to recruit and train a replacement. As a result of these protests the

Government allowed small employers a special privilege in this regard.

Section 56A states that s.56 shall not apply in relation to an employee if:

(a) *"immediately before the end of her maternity leave period (or, if it ends by reason of dismissal, immediately before the dismissal) the number of employees employed by her employer, added to the number employed by any associated employer of his did not exceed 5, and*

(b) *it is not reasonably practicable for the employer (who may be the same employer or a successor of his) to permit her to return to work in accordance with s.39, or for him or an associated employer to offer her employment under a contract of employment satisfying the conditions specified in ss.(3)".*

It is only the right to claim unfair dismissal that is excluded (and continues to be excluded after the recent amendments to this legislation) and if the reason for not reinstating the employee was a reason relating to redundancy then the employee would be entitled to claim a redundancy payment.

There is an exception to this — the small employer exception identified by the Employment Protection (Employment in Aided Schools) Order 1981, SI 1981/847 which applies to small state-aided schools. This is because although technically teachers are employed by school governors, they are in fact paid by local education authorities. This exception presumably arose since as the local education authority is the employer it should be able to find a supply teacher to cover the absence of a teacher.

Reorganisations

An employee is treated as not having been dismissed where "it is not practicable for a reason other than redundancy for the employer to permit her to return" in accordance with a s.39 of EP(C)A as substituted by TURERA 1993, s.23 (1)(b) Sch. 2 and an offer of suitable alternative employment is made to the employee and she accepts or unreasonably refuses that offer.

Suitable Alternative Employment

The small employers' exception only applies if it is not reasonably practicable to offer suitable alternative employment to the employee. Similarly, as already noted, the reorganisation exception only applies where an offer of suitable alternative employment is made and the employee either accepts or unreasonably refuses that offer.

The definition of suitable alternative employment in s.56A(3) is the same in both instances:

(a) the work to be done under the contract is of a kind which is both suitable in relation to the employee and appropriate for her to do in the circumstances, and

(b) the provisions of the contract as to the capacity and place in which she is to be employed and as to the other terms and conditions of her employment are not substantially less favourable to her than if she had returned to work under s.39 of the EP(C)A as substituted by TURERA 1993, s.23 (1)(b) Sch. 2.

Burden of Proof

The burden of proof is on the employer to show that either the small employers exception applies or that the reason for non-reinstatement was a reason other than redundancy and that no suitable alternative employment was available at the time. If the employer fails to discharge this burden of proof, then the dismissal is deemed to be automatically unfair.

Suspension Rights

TURERA 1993 will introduce a new right for pregnant women who are unable to continue working for health and safety reasons to be implemented by October 1994. Previously, an employer could fairly dismiss in such circumstances. This will no longer be the case. Section 22 will confer new rights on women to be suspended from work on grounds of maternity. Schedule 3 of the Act specifies these in detail (see Chapter 7 — Health and Safety).

Maternity Dismissals

Section 21 of TURERA 1993 amends s.60 of the EP(C)A and provides that all employees, regardless of their length of service or hours of service with the employer, have a right not to be dismissed on grounds of pregnancy or a pregnancy-related reason, or maternity or a reason related to maternity.

As a result of this provision, from 10 June 1994 employers are no longer able to fairly dismiss an employee on grounds that she is incapable of performing her job due to her pregnancy or because of a contravention of an enactment. No service qualification will be needed to bring a claim of unfair dismissal on grounds of pregnancy.

Automatically unfair dismissals

Section 60 as amended provides that the following reasons are now inadmissible reasons for dismissal.

- "The reason (or, if there is more than one, the principal reason) for her dismissal is that she is pregnant or any other reason connected with her pregnancy."

Therefore, it will automatically be unfair dismissal if an employee is dismissed because she is pregnant or for a pregnancy-related reason. This is the case even if she has only been employed for a couple of weeks.

- "Her maternity leave period is ended by the dismissal and the reason (or, if there is more than one, the principal reason) for her dismissal is that she has given birth to a child or any other reason connected with her having given birth to a child."

- "The reason (or, if there is more than one, the principal reason) for her dismissal, where her contract of employment was terminated after the end of her maternity leave period, is that she took, or availed, herself of the benefits of maternity leave."

This section is provided to protect an employee against victimisation by her employer.

- "The reason (or, if there is more than one, the principal reason for her dismissal) is that she has given birth to a child or any other reason connected with her having given birth to a child and before the end of her maternity leave period, she gave to her employer a certificate from a registered medical practitioner stating that by reason of disease or bodily or mental disablement she would be incapable of work after the end of that period and her contract of employment was terminated within the four week period following the end of her maternity leave period in circumstances where she continued to be incapable of work and the certificate relating to her incapacity remained current."
- "The reason (or, if there is more than one, the principal reason) for her dismissal is a requirement or recommendation such as is referred to in s.45(1), as substituted by TURERA 1993 s.25 Sch. 3."
- "Her maternity leave period is ended by the dismissal, and the reason (or, if there is more than one, the principal reason) for her dismissal is that she is redundant and s.38 as substituted by TURERA 1993 s.23(1)(a) has not been complied with." This will arise where an employer fails to offer suitable alternative employment to an employee who is made redundant while she is on short-term maternity leave.

Fair dismissal

It is still open to the employer to dismiss an employee on one of the grounds permitted by s.57. However, the burden is very much on the employer to show that the reason for dismissal fell within s.57(1), ie that the reason was one of those permitted by s.57(2) or "some other substantial reason of a kind such as to justify the dismissal of an employee holding the position which that employee held".

Section 57(2) sets out the reasons falling within s.57(1)(b) as follows. The dismissal was:

- related to the capability or qualifications of the employee for performing the work of the kind which she was employed by the employer to do, or

- related to the conduct of the employee, or
- the employee was redundant, or
- the employee could not continue to work in the position which she held without contravention (either on her part or on that of her employer) of a duty or restriction imposed by or under an enactment.

The general test of fairness is outlined in s.57(3) although it is slightly modified by s.2, paragraph 2(1) which is substituted for the general test set out in s.57(3). The schedule states that the determination of the question of whether the dismissal was either fair or unfair will depend on whether the employer would have been acting "reasonably or unreasonably in treating it as a sufficient reason for dismissing the employee if she had not been absent from work; and that question shall be determined in accordance with equity and the substantial merits of the case". This modification simply means that the employer on making redundancies whilst an employee is on maternity leave should consider her as though she were in fact still at work.

Automatic Right to Written Reasons for Dismissal

Section 53(2A) provides that, regardless of length of service, and employee is automatically entitled to receive a written statement giving the reasons for her dismissal if she is dismissed at any time whilst she is pregnant or after childbirth and during her maternity leave period. Normally, the right to such a written statement only arises if the employee has two years' continuous service and she has specifically requested such a statement. Section 53(2A) was incorporated into TURERA 1993 in order to comply with the EC Directive. Article 10(2) provides that if a pregnant worker, a worker who has recently given birth or a worker who is breast-feeding is dismissed during pregnancy or maternity leave, "the employer must cite duly substantiated grounds for her dismissal in writing".

The sanction for the employer should he or she fail to provide such a statement is to pay the employee two weeks' pay.

Figure 1: Notification of Maternity Leave/Resignation Due to Pregnancy

Surname	Forenames	Department	Payroll no.

Familiarise yourself with the statutory rights relating to maternity leave and maternity pay. (Leaflet can be obtained from the personnel department or the DSS and the Department of Employment.) Complete this form and return it to your supervisor as soon as possible but at least 21 days before starting maternity leave or leaving to have your baby.

This section to be completed by all employees.

1. I wish to confirm that I am *taking leave of absence/leaving work to have my baby. I will be stopping work on:
   (Please attach letter of resignation and notification of termination form where appropriate.)

   Day Month Year

2. My expected date of confinement is:

   Day Month Year

3. I enclose a copy of a certificate giving the expected date of my confinement issued by my *Doctor/Midwife: YES/NO
   This certificate will be returned to you.

This section to be completed only by those employees who are entitled to take maternity leave.

*4. I wish to confirm my intention to return to work after the birth of my baby and that I will return within the statutory period of 29 weeks beginning with the week in which my confinement falls.

*5. I do not wish to return to work after the birth of my baby.
   (Please attach letter of resignation and notification of termination form.)

Signature: _____   Date: _____

If you need further help or explanation, please contact:

_____

*Delete as appropriate

Figure 2: Maternity Leave

Surname	Forenames	Department	Payroll no.

Thank you for notifying us that you intend to take maternity leave and of your intention *not to/to return to work after the birth of your baby.

If you hold open your right to return to work you must:

1. Return to work within the statutory period allowed (within the period of 29 weeks beginning with the week in which your confinement falls); and

2. Write to us at least 21 days before the date you intend to return, giving us the precise date that you will start work again. (You may use the tear off slip below if you wish.)

We will write to you again during your maternity leave period to check whether you still wish to return to work. You *must* reply to that letter within 14 days of receiving it or you will lose the right to return.

Signature: _____ Date: _____

*Delete as appropriate

- -

Exercising the Right to Return to Work after Maternity Leave

To: _____ From: _____

I write to confirm that I shall be returning to work on the date below after taking maternity leave.

Day	Month	Year

Signature: _____ Date: _____

(This notification must be returned no later than 21 days before the date notified above and should be sent to your manager.)

Figure 3: Confirmation of Intention to Return to Work Following Maternity Leave

To: _____ From: _____

A. When notifying uf of your intention to take maternity leave, you indicated that you wished to return to work after the birth of your baby. As you are aware, this must be before the expiry of the statutory period of 29 weeks.

We are now writing to enquire whether or not you still intend to return to work.

Please send confirmation of this intention to us within 14 days of receipt of this correspondence or, if this is not possible, as soon as reasonably practicable. Failure to do this will lose you the right to return to work. You may use part C of this form for this purpose. Part B can be used to notify the actual date of return.

Signature: _____ Date: _____

B.   **Exercising the Right to Return to Work after Maternity Leave**

To: _____ From: _____

I write to confirm that I shall be returning to work on the date below after taking maternity leave.

Day	Month	Year

Signature: _____ Date: _____

(This notification must be returned not later than 21 days before the date above, and should be sent to your manager.)

C.   **Reply to Maternity Leave Confirmation Form**

To: _____ From: _____

*1. I wish to confirm my intention to return to work after my maternity leave and my date of return *is given below/will be sent to you in due course.

*2. I do not wish to return to work after my maternity leave.

Signature: _____ Date: _____

*Delete as appropriate

Question and Answers

Q: If an employee notifes me on her first day of work that she is pregnant, do I still have to give her paid leave?

A: *The employee's duty is to notify you at least 21 days before the expected week of the confinement or as soon as is reasonably practical. Her duty only arises as an employee and so if she tells you on her first day then you do have to give her the statutory 14 weeks' leave.*

Q: Does the employee have to give notice of her intention to return?

A: *Only when letting you know that she is going to take maternity leave. However if she is only going to take the 14 weeks' leave (all of it) she does not need to confirm her return date. If she has two years' service and is taking a longer period she must give notice.*

Q: What if the employee wants to come back early?

A: *The employee must give seven days' notice in writing and the employer can defer it by seven days. The Directive on which the new legislation in the UK is based requires Member States to provide for at least two weeks maternity leave to be compulsory.*

Q: What if she advises us that her child is sick?

A: *Unless you have specific provision in the employment contract (or it is your custom and practice to give special compassionate leave) then you would be entitled to advise her that she did not have the right to return. It is likely, however, that an employee will attempt to assert that this is sex discrimination on the same basis as is asserted in the case of Webb v Emo Air Cargo (UK) Ltd (see page 25).*

Q: Do I have to let the employee continue to use the company car during her maternity leave?

A: *Unless your company car policy has an express clause enabling you to require the return of that company car at any time and without cause which has been or would be exercised in other circumstances, then the* *answer to this question has to be yes. If the employee has more than two years' service at the relevant time and benefits from the 29 week post-natal time off right, then she will be entitled to the company car for the first 14 weeks but not (unless her contract of employment states otherwise) for the remaining 15 weeks! As a matter of practicality it would seem sensible to let the employee continue to use the company car for the entire period.*

Q: What if the employee is unable to work while she is pregnant because of Health and Safety Regulations?

A: *The new maternity provisions require you to, if possible, find her suitable alternative employment that does not involve any health and safety risk. Otherwise she is entitled to be paid on an ordinary basis but not to attend for work.*

Q: What if there are redundancies?

A: *An individual who has more than two years' service at the relevant time and is on maternity leave must be treated exactly the same as anyone else in relation to a redundancy situation. That means that she must be selected on a fair basis and on the same criteria as anybody else. Those criteria must be objective and rational and the individual on maternity leave should also be offered alternative work and should be consulted about the proposed redundancies in exactly the same way as any other employee. If the employee has less than two years' service and is on the 14 week period of maternity leave then there is no requirement for fair selection although there is a requirement to offer her any alternative job. You are not required to show an objective or fair redundancy selection so long as you can show that the pregnancy itself was not the reason for the selection.*

4 Redundancy

Introduction

Redundancy tends to be the most common reason for not allowing an employee to return to work following her maternity leave. The burden of proof is on the employer to show that the employee is genuinely redundant within the statutory definition of redundancy set out in s.81(2) EP(C)A 1978. This provides that:

> *"for the purposes of this Act an employee who is dismissed shall be taken to be dismissed by reason of redundancy if the dismissal is attributable wholly or mainly to:*
>
> *(a) the fact that her employer has ceased, or intends to cease, to carry on the business for the purposes of which the employee was employed by him, or has ceased, or intends to cease, to carry on that business in the place where the employee was so employed, or*
>
> *(b) the fact that the requirement of that business for employees to carry out work of a particular kind, or for employees to carry out work of a particular kind in the place where she was so employed, have ceased or diminished or are expected to cease or diminish or are expected to cease or diminish.*
>
> *For the purposes of this sub section, the business of the employer together with the business or businesses of his associated employers shall be treated as one unless either of the conditions specified in this sub section would be satisfied without so treating those businesses."*

If the employer fails to establish one of the grounds set out in s.81(2), then no reason for the employee's dismissal will have been established and her dismissal will be deemed automatically unfair.

Suitable Alternative Employment

Where there is a genuine redundancy situation, s.41(1), as substituted by TURERA s.23 (1)(b), Sch. 2, provides that an employee who qualifies for long-term maternity leave (or short-term maternity leave) and has a right to return to work at the end of her maternity leave period (ie has complied with the statutory notification requirements referred to in Chapter 3) will be treated as unfairly dismissed if she is not offered suitable alternative employment either with her employer or with an associated employer.

Failure to offer suitable alternative employment, if it is available, will mean that the dismissal is automatically unfair even if the employer has a reasonable excuse for the failure to make such an offer. For example, in *Community Task Force v Rimmer (1986) IRLR 203*, the EAT held that Mrs Rimmer should have been offered suitable alternative employment on another job creation scheme even though the MSC, which funded her employers, had threatened not to fund the project if the vacancy was offered to Mrs Rimmer in breach of MSC rules. The EAT pointed out that the test of availability under s.45(3) is not qualified by consideration of what is economic or reasonable and stress that if a suitable vacancy is available, it must be offered.

The burden is very much on the employer to find out whether suitable alternative employment is available and to offer it if it is available. In *John Menzies GB Ltd v Porter IRLB 457*, the EAT upheld an industrial tribunal's ruling that the company had failed in its statutory duty to offer alternative employment, even though the tribunal had not identified a vacant position. The EAT accepted that the industrial tribunal was entitled to conclude that the company had not made a proper effort to place Mrs Porter in a comparable position in another store and that such efforts it has made had been "half hearted and not co-ordinated".

Alternative Employment

Suitable alternative employment must be:

- suitable for the employee and appropriate for her to do in the circumstances, and

- such that the terms and conditions of the new contract as to the capacity and place in which she is to be employed as to the other terms of employment are not substantially less favourable to her than her old terms.

In broad terms, whether the work is suitable for the returner will be determined in the same way as suitable alternative employment is determined for redundancy purposes. Relevant factors will therefore include the status of the job, the place of work, travelling time, pay, hours and other conditions of work. Normally a job which is "suitable" will also be "appropriate", but is it possible that in considering the appropriateness of a particular position, a tribunal will take account of the particular circumstances of the employee and in particular her child care responsibilities, ie it may be incumbent on the employer to allow the returner to work flexible hours for a period of time. This may mean that the woman is in fact offered work which is more favourable to her than her original job.

Unreasonable Refusal of Offer by Employee

If an employee unreasonably refuses an offer of suitable alternative employment she will automatically lose her right to receive her redundancy payment and she will lose her statutory right to return.

Redundancy Entitlement

If there is no suitable alternative employment available, or if the employee is found to have reasonably turned down the offer of alternative employment, she will be entitled to a redundancy payment unless she is ineligible for such a payment for some other reason. An employee must normally submit her claim for a redundancy payment before the end of the six months from the NDR (s.101). That date is brought forward if the employer can show that she would have been made redundant earlier if she had not been on maternity leave.

Unfair Redundancies

Where there is a genuine redundancy situation, a dismissal may be unfair under Section 60 if the reason for dismissal is pregnancy or a reason connected with pregnancy, or is a reason connected with maternity leave.

Selection for redundancy must be based on fair and objective criteria and must not in any way relate to the fact that an employee is pregnant or absent on maternity leave. For example, in *Brown v Stockton on Tees Borough Council [1987] IRLR 263* the House of Lords held that an employee who was not offered alternative employment because she was pregnant and due to go on maternity leave had been dismissed for a reason connected with her pregnancy.

As far as procedural fairness is concerned, the fact that an employee is on maternity leave is no excuse for not consulting her. For example, in *John Menzies GB Ltd v Porter IRLB 457*, the industrial tribunal found that Mrs Porter's dismissal was unfair because of the "very worrying" procedural shortcomings. There had been no criteria for selecting those who were to be made redundant and there had been no prior consultation with Mrs Porter. On appeal the EAT agreed that the industrial tribunal was entitled to find that Mrs Porter's dismissal was unfair for this reason.

On the other hand, an employee on maternity leave is not entitled to preferential treatment although the burden is on the employer to show that her selection for redundancy would have been fair even if she had not been absent from work.

Short-term Maternity Leave

TURERA 1993 effectively extends these statutory provisions to those who are entitled to short-term maternity leave. The position regarding those on short-term maternity leave may therefore be summarised as follows.

- Employees who become redundant during the 14 week maternity leave period have a right to be offered suitable alternative employment.

- The dismissal of employees who are not offered suitable alternative employment will be automatically unfair.

- The dismissal of an employee on, or prior to, short-term maternity leave will be automatically unfair if the reason for dismissal is in any way connected with pregnancy or their period of maternity leave. However, their selection for redundancy will not be unfair if these factors are ignored.

- In theory, employees who are unfairly selected for redundancy during the maternity leave period cannot complain of unfair dismissal as they do not qualify for protection against unfair dismissal under the ordinary rules. However, where an employee is unfairly selected there is a danger that an industrial tribunal will draw an inference that they have been unfairly selected for an inadmissible reason, namely pregnancy or maternity.

- Employees who become redundant while they are on short-term maternity leave should be consulted before they are dismissed.

- Employees on short-term maternity leave will not be entitled to a redundancy payment as they do not qualify for such payments under the statutory provisions.

Implementing Redundancies

The question of the date on which an employee who becomes redundant during maternity leave should actually be regarded as dismissed is not entirely resolved. Section 86, as amended states that:

"Where an employee is entitled to return to work and has exercised her right to return in accordance with s.47 (has the right to return under s.39 and has exercised it in accordance with s.42) but is not permitted to return to work, then she shall be treated for the purpose of the provisions of this part as if she had been employed until the notified day of return, and, if she would not otherwise be so treated, as having been continuously employed until that day, and as if she had been dismissed with effect from that day for the reason for which she was not permitted to return."

Under paragraph 5 of Sch.2, however, if the employer shows that the reason for his or her failure to let the employee return is that the employee is redundant and was dismissed, or would have been dismissed had she continued to be employed by him or her by reason of redundancy on a day during her maternity absence.

Paragraph 5 says:

"For the purposes of Part VI of this Act the employee:

(1) shall not be treated as having been dismissed with effect from the notified date of return but

(2) shall, if she would not otherwise be so treated, be treated as having been continuously employed until that earlier day and as having been dismissed by reason of redundancy with effect from that day."

The wording of s.45, substituted by TURERA 1993, s.41, also suggests that a redundancy can be carried out before the notified day of return.

It is clear then that the employee has a right to a redundancy payment at the time of the actual redundancy. However, it seems that the wording of the return to work provisions also mean that there is, in essence, a continuing obligation upon the employer to look out for alternative work pending the notified date of return and that she has a right to return to work.

Probably the safest course for an employer who may need to make redundant a woman on maternity leave is commence discussions with that individual prior to making the final selection of employees for redundancy. These discussions should alert her to the potential redundancy and indicate that the nature of the selection criteria being adopted means that she is likely to be one of those who is selected for redundancy. After selection has been carried out and the individual has been declared redundant, a redundancy payment should be made to them at the same time as it is made to other staff. The redundancy date should be such that notice is received prior to it in accordance with the employee's contract. The employee should be invited for further consultations upon confirmation of her redundancy and should be advised to notify her employer of her intended date of return, in relation to alternative employment, and up to that date the situation should be kept under review to decide whether or not there is a suitable alternative vacancy for her.

Notice Payments

Employees on short-term maternity leave are entitled to notice pay if they are made redundant prior to their return from maternity leave. The position is less clear regarding those on long-term maternity leave. If the redundancy takes effect prior to the employee's return to work, then on the face of it she is not entitled to notice pay over and above her maternity pay, during that period. Schedule 3, which protects individuals who are off sick during their notice period, does not cover maternity pay and therefore there does not seem to be any express provision regarding payment of notice to a woman on maternity leave. However it is arguable that if the contract is merely suspended during the period of maternity leave (see page 47) that the rights of those on long-term maternity leave to notice pay are preserved. Furthermore, if other staff are being paid monies in lieu of notice, it may be a matter of fairness that a woman on maternity leave should also be paid such notice. She may also have an argument in relation to the Sex Discrimination Act 1975 (based on the *Dekker* and *Hertz* decisions) in this situation.

Repayment of Redundancy Monies

Paragraph 6(4) of Schedule 2 provides for repayment of a redundancy payment made to a woman on maternity leave if alternative employment is subsequently found for her and if the employer requests such repayment. The employer would be advised as a precaution to expressly reserve the right to recover the payment in these circumstances at the time payment is made, since the final words of paragraph 6(4)(b) says; "if the employer requests such a repayment". Also, such a proviso will provide evidence that the employer was genuinely trying to find the employee alternative work, should this be challenged.

Questions and Answers

Q: How should I consult with a woman on maternity leave about redundancy?

A: *Prior to selection you should write informing her of the potential redundancies and that the selection criteria mean that she is likely to be selected. The letter should also invite her to discuss with you the potential redundancy and the possibility of alternative employment. Upon selection a further letter should be issued informing her of her likely dismissal and inviting her to a further consultation session to discuss alternative employment. The employee should also be advised to notify you of the date on which she would wish to return to alternative employment and up to that date you should continue to look out for alternative vacancies for her and consult with her over any possibilities that occur. At the end of that period if no vacancies have been found she should be invited for a final consultation.*

Q: If, objectively, she is the person who should be selected can she be dismissed for redundancy?

A: *Yes, a pregnant woman can still be made redundant for reasons unconnected with her pregnancy, provided she has been fairly selected and her selection is not in any way due to her pregnancy. She can be dismissed during her confinement at the same time as any of her colleagues who are also redundant (as long as the notice requirements in her contract and the consultation requirements explained above are complied with).*

Q: Do I still have to keep her in mind for other jobs?

A: *Yes, although she can be dismissed for redundancy during her maternity leave the obligation on you to look out for alternative employment continues until the date on which the employee would return to work if such employment were available.*

Q: Is she entitled to notice pay?

A: *On the face of it she has no entitlement to full pay during her notice period if she is on maternity leave. There are no statutory provisions entitling her to notice pay. However where other employees are receiving pay in lieu of notice she may have a claim under the SDA that she has received unfavourable treatment due to her confinement if she does not receive notice pay.*

5 Maternity Pay

Introduction

The Maternity Allowance and Statutory Maternity Pay Regulations 1994 ("the Regulations") were introduced on 4 May 1994. The Regulations amend the Social Security Contributions and Benefits Act 1992 so as to either implement the requirements detailed in the Council Directive 92/85/EEC in relation to allowances made to women on maternity leave or to enable such requirements to be implemented in subordinate legislation made under that Act.

There are two types of maternity pay available to eligible pregnant employees:

- Statutory Maternity Pay (SMP), and
- Maternity Allowance (MA).

SMP is paid by the employer to the employee and MA is paid by the DSS to those employees not eligible to receive SMP. SMP is paid at two rates: a higher rate and a lower rate (see page 95).

The system by which employers pay maternity benefits to employees underwent substantial changes when the Social Security Act 1986 was brought into force on 6 April 1987. A revised Maternity Pay Scheme called Statutory Maternity Pay was introduced under this legislation.

Maternity Allowance

MA is available to pregnant women who are not "employees" (ie employed persons who for some reason do not qualify for SMP, self-employed persons or casuals). It is a weekly benefit payable for a maximum of 18 weeks direct from the DSS. Responsibility for the payment of MA lies with the Department of Social Security.

Eligibility

In order to be eligible for MA the pregnant woman:

- must have either reached or been confined before reaching the commencement of the 11th week before the EWC, and
- must have been engaged in employment as an employed or self-employed earner for at least 26 weeks in the 66 weeks ending with the week before the expected week of confinement, and
- must not be entitled to SMP, and
- must satisfy the specified contribution conditions.

In effect, this means that sufficient Class 1 or Class 2 NIC must have been paid in respect of at least 26 weeks in the period of 66 weeks ending with the week before the EWC. This period is referred to as the "test period".

NIC paid by the employed earner or the self-employed earner must have been either full-rate Class 1 or Class 2 contributions.

How to Claim MA

If an employee who has claimed SMP is either not entitled to receive SMP or has become disentitled then the employer is obliged to provide her with a completed DSS form SMP1 together with any maternity certificate MATB1 signed by her midwife or doctor which she may have already given to the employer. On this form the employer must state the reasons for not paying SMP to the employee. This should be dealt with within seven days of the employer having decided that an employee is not eligible to receive SMP. The employee will then be in a position to hand the form to her local Social Security Office to claim MA.

If the woman is either not employed during the 15th week before the EWC or she is self-employed, the claim is made on the DSS claim form MA1 which, once completed, should be sent to the local Social Security Office together with a medical certificate detailing the expected date of the birth. (If she is working, form SMP1 must also be submitted stating why she is not entitled to SMP.) The form may still be submitted even if the woman is not at that stage in possession of the requisite medical evidence.

Payment of MA

MA cannot be paid before the beginning of the 11th week before the EWC. It is paid for a period of up to 18 weeks, referred to as the Maternity Allowance Period (MAP).

Unless the birth is premature, the MAP must always include a "core period" of 13 weeks which commences six weeks before the expected birth. The remainder of the MAP may be taken either before or after the "core period".

The MAP cannot commence earlier than five weeks before the "core period", which in effect means not before the 11th week before the EWC. In addition, the MAP cannot start later than the beginning of the core period (ie six weeks before the EWC).

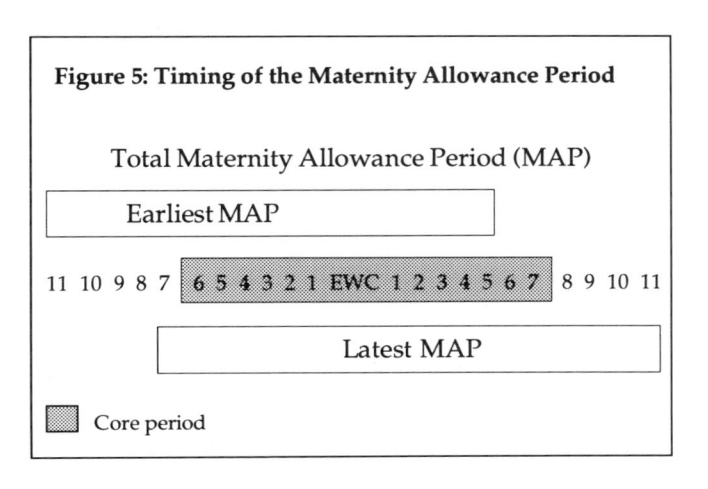

Figure 5: Timing of the Maternity Allowance Period

Total Maternity Allowance Period (MAP)

Earliest MAP

11 10 9 8 7 6 5 4 3 2 1 EWC 1 2 3 4 5 6 7 8 9 10 11

Latest MAP

▨ Core period

MA is not payable whilst the employee continues working. Therefore, if the employee continues to work into the core period she will not receive her full 18 weeks' entitlement. MA is paid from the day the employee stops work.

If the birth takes place later than expected, the MAP nevertheless remains the same although if the woman remains unable to return to work, she may be entitled to claim Sickness Benefit. If a woman has exhausted her entitlement to both MA and Sickness Benefit, she may be able to claim Invalidity Benefit.

Amount Payable

An employee employed in the week immediately preceding the 14th week before the EWC, shall receive a weekly rate equal to the lower rater of SMP, currently £52.50.

Employees who are self-employed or who have recently become unemployed shall receive a weekly rate of £45.55.

Checklist: Maternity Allowance

- Payable to employees not eligible for SMP.

- Payable for up to 18 weeks.

- Payable to employees who have worked and paid NIC for at least 26 weeks in the 66 weeks immediately before the week before the EWC.

- Employer to provide employee with a completed SMP1 and maternity certificate (if in his or her possession) within seven days of having decided that the employee is not eligible for SMP.

- MA not liable to income tax and NIC.

Statutory Maternity Pay

The right to receive SMP is contingent upon the employee satisfying a number of conditions relating to her employment. If any of the conditions are not fulfilled then the employee is not entitled to receive SMP although, as discussed above, she may instead be able to claim Maternity Allowance from the State.

SMP is payable at two rates, the higher rate and the lower rate.

There is no requirement for a written contract of employment to exist provided the employer pays NIC.

Eligibility

To be eligible for SMP an employee must fulfil the following conditions:

- she must have been continuously employed by her employer for at least 26 weeks continuing into the 15th week before the EWC — this 15th week is known as the Qualifying Week (QW)
- she must have stopped working for the employer wholly or partly as a result of the pregnancy or confinement
- her average weekly earnings must not be less than the lower earnings limit (LEL) in force at the time for payment of NIC for the period of eight weeks ending with the QW
- she must have become pregnant and still be pregnant at the beginning of the 11th week before the EWC, or have given birth at that time
- she must give 21 days' notice to her employer that she intends to stop work because of pregnancy; or as soon as is reasonably practicable
- she must produce medical evidence of her EWC.

Calculating the Qualifying Week

The QW is the 15th week before the EWC. The EWC is simply the week in which the birth is expected to take place. The expected date of confinement (EDC) will be identified on the maternity certificate or such other appropriate medical document.

It is important to note that "week" in this context refers to the period of seven days beginning with a Sunday and ending on a Saturday; it is of no significance that the employee's pay week may span a different seven day period. The employment must have commenced before the Sunday which commences before the 15th week before the EWC.

Therefore the employee must be employed into the 15th week before the EWC. It is not necessary for the employee to be employed for the whole of that 15th week as long as she is employed for at least part of that week.

It is interesting to note that an employee will be regarded as employed so long as her contract of employment continues into the QW. Therefore, it is of no significance that the employee did not actually work into the QW so long as the employment contract exists until that time.

Typically there are however a number of exceptions to this general rule.

- Where an employer brings a contract of employment to an end for the purpose of avoiding liability for SMP he or she is liable to make payments of SMP to any woman who has been continuously employed for at least eight weeks. The employee is deemed to have been employed until the QW.

- To determine the amount due to the employee, she shall be treated as having been employed from the date of her employment with that employer, until the end of the week immediately preceding the 14th week before the EWC, on the same terms and conditions as those which had existed before her employment was terminated. The normal weekly earnings for the period of eight weeks immediately preceding the 14th week before the EWC is calculated by reference to the employee's normal weekly earnings for the period of eight weeks ending with the last day on which she was paid under her former contract of employment. Therefore, an employer cannot escape liability.

- Provision is made for a woman to be treated as having been continuously employed where she is confined before the QW and gives birth to a live child. It simply needs to be ascertained that the woman would have been continuously employed up to the QW if she had not gone into early confinement and that her normal weekly earnings for the eight weeks preceding the week of confinement were not below the LEL.

Agency Workers

The liability for payment of SMP to agency workers rests with their employing agency if the employee has 26 weeks' continuous service in the QW.

The continuity of service is not broken if the woman is absent from work during the 26 week period as a result of sickness, injury, pregnancy or due to the agency not being able to offer the woman work at that particular time. However, the entitlement to SMP is based on the proviso that the woman will return to work after the period of absence.

If the employee was not employed in the QW, she can still be treated as though she was employed in that week if:

- the employing agency had no available work to offer the woman in that week, and
- the woman was not intending to commence her maternity leave at that particular time and was always available for work after the QW as soon as the agency were able to find something for her, and
- the woman does, in fact, have further employment with the agency before commencing her maternity leave.

As long as an employee carries out some work during any week, then that is treated as a full week, when her continuity of employment is being computed.

If in any week the agency was not able to provide an employee with work, her continuity is not broken.

If she was offered work but was unable to perform it, that period of absence can only count towards continuity if she was unavailable due to her pregnancy or sickness or injury. If the reason for the unavailability was sickness then the employee must resume work with the agency within 26 weeks.

Should the employee have actually stopped looking for work through a particular agency before the QW, then the agency is not liable to pay the higher rate SMP.

The same notification requirements apply to agency workers as to normal employees.

Seasonal or Regular Casual Workers

Certain businesses require casual workers and employ seasonal staff. Obviously due to the nature of their employment such employees experience breaks in their service since they only work as and when required. Employees who undertake employment of this nature do not necessarily break their continuity of employment as a result of such breaks so long as it can be demonstrated that the break has only been of a "temporary" nature.

In the case of *Ford v Warwickshire County Council (1983) ICR 273* Lord Diplock stated that the words "temporary" meant lasting for only a relatively short period of time and that it was necessary to apply what has become known as the "mathematical" approach to ascertain whether the interval between the two contracts was short in relation to the combined duration. Additionally, in the case of *Flack and Others v Kodak Ltd (1986) ICR 775* it was stated that all the relevant circumstances should be taken into account and in particular the length of the period of absence should be considered in the context of the period of employment as a whole.

However, the fact that the employer intends to re-employ the applicant after the break in the employment does not necessarily indicate that there was only a temporary cessation of work in the sense of being for a relatively short period of time — *Sillars v Charringtons Fuels Ltd (1989) ICR 475*.

In *Lloyds Bank Ltd v Secretary of State of Employment (1979) IRLR 41* it was held that working alternate weeks during a year not break the continuity of employment where the absence was by reason of "custom or arrangement". The contract of employment in this case was regarded as continuing even during the weeks in which the employee was absent.

The scope of "arrangement or custom" was widened by the SMP (General) Amendment Regulations 1990 in order to benefit more employees whose employment was of a spasmodic nature. The Regulations state that in order for employees with employment of this seasonal and temporary nature to ensure the preservation of their continuity of employment, the following conditions must be satisfied:

- the employer customarily offers the employee work for a fixed period of not more than 26 weeks, and
- such offers of employment are made to the employee on two or more occasions in any one year for periods which do not overlap, and
- the offers of employment are made to employees who had worked for that employer during the last or recent period when that type of employment was required.

If these above conditions are satisfied then, even if the employee is absent in the QW either wholly or partly because of pregnancy or confinement or as a result of disease or disablement, continuity of employment is preserved as regards eligibility for SMP. This is the case even if the employee fails to return to work before her maternity leave begins.

Change of Employer

The continuity of employment provision states that employment must be with the same employer. However, there are certain circumstances where continuity of employment is preserved despite there having been a change of employer.

- There is a transfer of the employer's trade business or undertaking to another.

    The new employer assumes the role of the previous employer and so the employee's continuity of employment is preserved — Transfer of Undertakings (Protection of Employment) Regulations 1981, Regulation 5. However, if these regulations do not apply then the new employer takes over and new contracts are commenced between the new employer and the employees. In those circumstances, no continuity is preserved and the new employer has no responsibility for the payment of SMP and the employee has to start again as regards accumulating time for entitlement to the various statutory maternity rights.

- Where under an Act of Parliament, a contract of employment between any body corporate and the employee is modified and some other body corporate is substituted as her employer.
- Where on the death of her employer, the employee is taken into the employment of the personal representatives or trustees of the deceased.
- Where the employee is employed by partners, personal representatives or trustees and there is a change in the partners, personal representatives or trustees.
- Where the employee is taken into the employment of another employer who is, at the time an "associated employer" of her previous employer.
- Where on the termination of her employment with a school maintained by a local education authority the employee is taken into the employment of another employer maintained by the same local education authority including schools where the governors of that school are the employers (rather than the local education authority).

Continuity is also preserved where an employee re-enters her employment after not more than six months away with the reserve service of the armed forces. The period of absence does not, however, count in computing her period of continuous employment.

Average Weekly Earnings

In order for an employee to be entitled to SMP (either the higher or lower rate), her average weekly earnings for the period of eight weeks ending with the last payday immediately preceding the end of the QW must be at or above the lower earnings limit (LEL) for the payment of NIC. There is no upper limit of weekly earnings. The LEL is currently £57.00 per week.

Calculation of Average Weekly Earnings

There are three methods by which an employer can calculate the average weekly earnings. The appropriate method depends upon whether the employee is paid on a weekly basis, a monthly basis or at other intervals.

It is important to remember that when calculating the average weekly earnings, it is the employee's actual earnings during the relevant eight week period which should be used for the computation.

Weekly paid employees

Take the employee's earnings for the last eight paydays ending with the last payday before the end of the QW and divide that figure by eight.

Figure 6: Last Eight Paydays before the End of the End of the QW

1	2	3	4	5	6	7	8
£70	£70	£110	£130	£80	£100	£50	£50

Total £660 ÷ 8 = <u>£82.50</u>

The resulting figure is the employee's average weekly earnings. All payments in the eight calendar weeks prior to the QW must be included. Therefore if, for example the employee has been paid in advance for a holiday and so was not due any payment on one of the paydays, that week must still be included in the calculations.

Monthly paid employees

The gross payment on the last payday on or before the end of the QW should be added to any other payments made after but not including the earlier payday which fell at least eight weeks before the last payday. That total should then be multiplied by six and divided by 52. The resulting figure gives the average weekly earnings.

Employees paid monthly but in multiples of a week

Take the gross payment made on the last payday before the end of the QW and any other payments made after, but not including, the last payday which fell at least eight weeks before that date. That amount is then divided by the number of weeks covered by those payments.

Employees paid at other intervals

Add together the gross payment on the last day before the end of the QW and any other payments made after, but including, the last payday that fell at least eight weeks earlier than the last payday. Therefore the period over which the earnings are averaged begins on the day after the earlier payday and ends with the last payday before the QW. If the number of days in this period is an exact number of weeks namely divisible by seven then the figure should be divided by the number of weeks. If the period is not an exact number of weeks, the relevant earnings should be divided by the number of days in that period and then multiplied by seven. The result is the average weekly earnings.

These methods of calculating the average weekly earnings cover the "normal" maternity situation. However, the method of calculation is different if the employee gives birth before the end of the QW and it is a live birth.

To calculate such an employee's average weekly earnings the employer would take the last payday before the week of confinement and substitute this payday as the base date rather than the last payday before the end of the QW. The average weekly earnings are then calculated using the appropriate method out of those mentioned above. In this case an employee will only be entitled to SMP if she would have been entitled had she remained in employment until the QW.

Aggregation of Earnings

It is possible for an employee who works under more than one contract for the same employer or associated employer (where the employer aggregates the gross wages for each contract for the purposes of NIC) to aggregate her hours for the purposes of calculating SMP entitlement. In the same way, she is also entitled to aggregate her earnings under both contracts and thereby treat the earnings from each employment as if they had all been paid by the last employer in the period, for the purposes of calculating her average weekly earnings.

Therefore, if NIC under each contract are dealt with separately then an employee's eligibility for SMP must also be dealt with separately and the eligibility must be calculated separately. In addition, if an employee works under more than one contract but the employers are not the same and are not associated, then obviously an employee is not entitled to aggregate either her hours worked or her earnings since the liability for repayment of NIC lies with each employer individually.

Where an employee is involved in more than one contract with the same employer, they are to be treated "as one".

Pregnant at the 11th Week Before EWC

An employee must actually still be pregnant at the 11th week before her EWC or alternatively have given birth to a live child before that date.

If the birth takes place exceptionally early, namely before the 15th week before the EWC, the continuous service rule will nevertheless still be satisfied if the employee, but for her early confinement, would have been in employment for a continuous period of at least 26 weeks at the QW and if her average weekly earnings are calculated with reference to the eight weeks ending with the week before the week in which she gave birth.

If reasonably practicable, the employee should provide notice of the date of the birth within 21 days.

Notification of Maternity Absence

An employee must notify her employer that she is going to be absent from work on account of her pregnancy or confinement. Failure to do so will disqualify her from receiving SMP.

The employee must normally give at least 21 days' notice before her absence is due to begin or if this is not "reasonably practicable", as soon as it is reasonably practicable.

Means of Giving Notice

The means of giving notice does not have to be in writing unless the employer so requests but it does have to be in writing for the statutory right to return so it may be best to specify that notice should be given in writing. It is the employer's responsibility to decide how he or she wishes to be notified and employees should be advised of this.

Failure to Give Requisite Notice

If the employee does not provide the employer with at least 21 days' notice, it is the employer's responsibility to decide whether or not it was "reasonably practicable" for her to have given such notice and whether or not her lack of notification means that she loses her entitlement to SMP.

Aggrieved Employee

If the employer decides that the employee is not entitled to SMP as a result of the lack of or late notification, the employee is entitled to ask the employer to provide her with a written statement of the reasons for refusal. If the employee is still not satisfied once she has read the employer's statement, the employee may appeal against the decision and refer the matter to a DSS Adjudication Officer (see Chapter 6).

Exceptions to the Notification Requirement

There are two specific situations where an employee is exempt from the requirement to give 21 days' notice before commencing maternity leave. They are as follows:

- if the employee leaves her employment for a reason wholly unconnected with her pregnancy after the beginning of the QW, or

- if the employee is dismissed before having given notice that she is going to be absent from work because of pregnancy or confinement.

However the employer must still be given notice of the actual date of confinement if the employee is confined before the 11th week before the QW. Since the MPP would normally start with the 11th week, if the employee is confined earlier than the EWC then the MPP begins with the week following the week of confinement and so obviously the employer needs to know when this is.

It would be advisable for the employer to inform all employees of this 21 days' notice requirement and confirm with an employee the actual date when notice should be given.

Additional Notice Requirement

There are two special cases where an employee having already given the proper notice of her impending absence is also obliged to give additional notice to her employer. The situations are as follows.

- Where the employee is confined during or before the QW:
    - the employee must give notice to the employer that her absence is "wholly because of her confinement"
    - this notice must be given within 21 days of the date she was confined or if that is not practicable as soon as is reasonably practicable thereafter
    - the notice must be in writing if so requested by the employer.

- Where the employee has previously given notice of her impending absence as required but is subsequently confined before the scheduled date of absence:
    - the employee is obliged to provide a further notice for the employer "specifying the date she was confined and the date of her absence"

- this notice must be given within 21 days of the actual day of confinement although if it is not practicable to do so then it should be done as soon as is reasonably practicable
- the notice must be in writing if so requested by the employer.

In the above circumstances "a notice contained in an envelope which is properly addressed and sent by prepaid post shall be deemed to be given on the date on which it is posted". This provision only applies to the situations described above and not to the normal 21 days' notice of impending absence.

Medical Evidence

An employee is obliged to provide an employer with medical evidence of the EWC or of the date she was actually confined.

The employee must provide the employer with a Maternity Certificate (MATB1) which must be issued by a doctor or a registered midwife.

The certificate must contain:

- the employee's name
- the EWC or the actual date of confinement if the certificate is issued after the confinement and the EDC is later than the date of the actual confinement
- the examination date which led to the production of the medical certificate
- the date the certificate was signed, and
- the address of the doctor who signed the certificate or if signed by a registered midwife his or her registered number or address.

The maternity certificate is essential in order for the employer to be able to calculate an employee's entitlement to SMP. An employer may obtain a maternity certificate from a local DSS office which he or she may then request the employee to have completed by a doctor or midwife.

The medical certificate must be submitted to the employer no later than the third week of the maternity pay period although the employer may accept evidence of the EDC later if he or she accepts the employee's reasons for not having previously provided it. However, in no circumstances can medical evidence be provided later than the end of the 13th week of the MPP.

An employee who provides an inadequate medical certificate may be disqualified from receiving SMP. However this does not disqualify her from her statutory right to return to work.

Checklist: Notification of Maternity Absence

- 21 days' notice of intention to take maternity leave is required.

- Notice should be written if the employer so requests.

- Medical certificate giving the EWC to be submitted no later than the third week of the MPP (unless the employee can shown good reason for the lateness).

- Notification of change of circumstances which may affect entitlement to SMP is required (see below).

Rates of SMP

SMP is payable to eligible employees at two rates, namely the higher rate and the lower rate.

Higher Rate

The higher rate is a weekly rate equivalent to 90% of the employee's "normaly weekly earnings" for the period of eight weeks immediately preceding the 14th week before the EWC or the current weekly Statutory Sick Pay entitlement, whichever is higher. The higher rate is payable to eligible employees for a period of six weeks.

Lower Rate

The Lower Rate is currently £52.50 and is payable for the remaining 12 weeks of the Maternity Pay Period (MPP).

Change in Circumstances

There is an obligation to notify an employer of a change in circumstances which may affect employee's entitlement to SMP:

- **Engaged in work for another employer.**

    If, after an employee's confinement, she undertakes work for another employee, the original employer's liability to pay SMP ceases. The liability stops on the Saturday of the week preceding the week during which she starts work for someone else.

- **Employee goes outside the EEA.**

    SMP is not payable for any week during which the employee is outside the EEA. The employer's liability ceases at the end of the last complete week before she goes outside the EEA. The employer should give employee form SMP1 and her maternity certificate as she may be able to claim a state benefit.

- **Employee taken into legal custody.**

    An employer's liability to pay SMP ceases when an employee is taken into legal custody, namely detained, arrested or imprisoned. The employee is not disqualified if she is voluntarily assisting the police. The employer should provide the employee with her form SMP1 and her maternity certificate in order that she may apply for a State benefit instead.

The Maternity Pay Period

The Maternity Pay Period (MPP) is the period during which Statutory Maternity Pay (SMP) is payable to an eligible employee. SMP is payable to an eligible employee for 18 consecutive weeks.

The MPP cannot commence earlier than the 11th week before the EWC but apart from this restriction an employee can delay the commencement of the MPP until the week immediately following the week in which she is confined. Effectively, an employer has no right to force an employee to leave work to commence her maternity leave at a particular time although one must remember the exception to this "freedom to in choose" which was referred to earlier in chapter 3, page 36, where a woman is absent from work in the six weeks, prior to the EWC wholly or partly due to pregnancy.

Employee who Works after MPP has Begun

If an employee's MPP has commenced and the employee decides to engage in some work for her employer in any week or part of a week, then she will lose her entitlement to SMP for that week. If an employee does work during a week in which she is eligible for the higher rate of SMP, she will lose that week's entitlement at the lower rate and not at the higher rate.

An employee will therefore have to weigh up her financial position in order to decide whether to work during her MPP and receive her regular salary against losing her right to receive SMP (at the lower rate) in respect of each week for which she works once the MPP has begun.

Working for Another Employer during the MPP

It is of no significance and therefore does not affect an employee's entitlement to SMP if, during her MPP but before the birth of her child, she undertakes work for another employer who is not liable to pay her SMP.

The employer who employed her at the qualifying week (QW) will still be liable to pay the SMP.

However, if an employee works during the MPP but after the baby is born, that will end the original employer's liability to pay her SMP for the remainder of the MPP from the Saturday of the week in which she commenced work with another employer.

There is a duty on the employee to inform her original employer if she should commence work for another employer during that MPP.

However, if the employee worked for more than one employer during the qualifying week but one of them is liable to pay her SMP, then she is entitled to remain working for the non-SMP liable employer throughout the MPP even though she receives SMP from the liable employer.

Employment Terminates after the QW

If the employee resigns or is fairly dismissed after the QW, SMP payments will be paid in the normal manner.

Birth before the Start of the MPP

In these circumstances, MPP will commence the week after the week in which the birth occurred.

Events which may Disentitle the Employee from SMP

There are a number of situations which may occur during the MPP which may disentitle an employee from receiving SMP.

- **If the employee is placed in legal custody or sentenced to imprisonment.**
  An employee automatically loses her entitlement to SMP. The only exception here is if she is given a suspended sentence of imprisonment.

  If this occurs during the first week of the MPP then an employee loses her right to SMP completely.

Regulations clearly state that an employee is not liable to any SMP for any week within the MPP or any part of which she is so detained and for any subsequent week within that period. Therefore, an employee in such a situation loses her right to SMP with effect from that particular week. It is the employee's responsibility to inform an employer that she has been taken into legal custody.

- **If an employee is outside the European Economic Area.**
  Entitlement to SMP will stop with effect from the first week in which an employee is outside the EEA. Obviously, if an employee is simply in transit between two Member States then she is not treated as being outside the EEA.

- **The death of an employee during her MPP.**
  The death of an employee during her MPP automatically terminates the employer's liability to make payments of SMP in respect of any week within the MPP which falls after the week in which the death occurred. There is no provision for claims in respect of outstanding SMP on behalf of the deceased employee's estate.

- **The employee undertaking work during the MPP.**
  This is matter has already been addressed earlier in this chapter but in brief, an employee loses her entitlement to SMP for any week during which she works for her employer. But she is only disentitled for the week in which she has actually performed some work.

Payment and Administration of SMP

Deductions

SMP is to be regarded as "earnings" for social security purposes. The employer should therefore deduct PAYE income tax and national insurance contributions (NIC) and any other deductions as though it were pay. The employers must also of course account for their own share of NIC. Therefore, any deductions that can lawfully be made from pay can equally be made from SMP.

Off-setting

Certain *contractual payments* to an employee may be offset against SMP or vice versa including:

- contractual pay which an employer pays to an employee who is no longer at work
- contractual sick pay
- contractual maternity pay.

Therefore, if any of the above contractual payments are made during the MPP such payments can be treated as either reducing or extinguishing the liability to SMP for that week or alternatively the employer can pay SMP in the normal manner and simply withhold a corresponding sum from any of the relevant contractual payments outlined above.

Manner of Payment

There are actually no specific provisions dealing with the timing and manner of payment of SMP.

In making the payment, employers may follow their normal payroll practice although, where there is no normal practice, the remuneration should be paid on the last day of a calendar month.

Lump Sum

Employers are often tempted to pay the SMP in a lump sum to an employee who in effect has no employment protection since she has not worked for a continuous period of two years up to the 11th week before the EWC. The reasoning behind this is that the employee can be taken off the books and there is no further administrative work in relation to her. This was a more straightforward means of paying under the old SMP scheme, however the payment of a lump sum under the present scheme may cause problems for the employer. Under the current SMP provisions there are a number of ways in which an employee may lose her entitlement to SMP during the MPP. For example, as discussed earlier, entitlement is lost if an employee goes abroad outside the EC. In such a situation, if the employer has paid SMP entitlement in a lump sum the employer then has to consider how to recover the overpayment. It may not be possible to recover that amount from the DSS and if the employee herself refuses to repay the overpayment the employer will have to take the requisite legal action against the employee in order to recover it.

In addition, tax and NIC are payable on the SMP and if payment is made as a lump sum it will be treated as earnings in the period in which it is paid which could obviously make a difference to the amount payable by both the employer and employee. In effect the amount of NIC payable will be more on a lump sum payment than if the employee was paid on either a weekly or monthly basis.

Employee Unable/Incapable of Acting on Her Own Behalf

If it is evident that the employee is unable to act on her own behalf, the employer could make arrangements for the payments to be made instead to another person such as, for example, her next of kin. If the employer is unaware of any suitable person to make the payments to then he or she is best advised to contact the local DSS office which will deal with the matter.

Recovery of SMP by the Employer and NIC Compensation

With effect from 4 September 1994 employers can recover an amount equal to 92% of SMP payable in a tax month to eligible employees (although "small employers" will continue to receive full reimbursement). This is done by deducting the amount paid from the total amount of NIC and tax paid to the Inland Revenue every month.

It is largely up to the employer as to how he or she times the recovery. The employer is entitled to deduct the payments from his or her income tax contributions for the tax month in which the SMP was paid but not for those for any earlier month. This recovery may also be made from later contributions provided they are made before six years after the tax year in which the SMP was paid.

An employer may well find that the SMP paid actually exceeds the total NIC due in a particular month. If this is the case, the excess amount of SMP may be deducted from the PAYE income tax due for that month. If the excess is more than *both* the NIC and income tax due in a particular month then the employer should carry the excess forward and deduct the amount from payments due in the subsequent month.

If the recovery of the excess is needed more quickly then the employer may write to the Inland Revenue Accounts office to see how the problem can be resolved.

Mistakes

If a mistake is made in respect of SMP payments the employer should rectify it immediately.

SMP1 Issued By Mistake

If an employer discovers that an SMP1 form has been issued in error and that the employee was entitled to receive SMP, the employer should do the following.

- Contact the employee to inform her of her entitlement.
- Contact the appropriate Social Security office in order to avoid State benefit being paid in error. If the employer does not know which Social Security office to contact, he or she should simply contact his or her own office and they will pass the information on to the correct office.
- Pay the SMP to the employee.

SMP Wrongly Paid/Too Much Paid

The employer should immediately contact the local Social Security office if payment has been made when an employee was not in fact entitled to receive it. On informing the Social Security office, the employer will be requested to complete a form so that the employee concerned can then claim a Social Security benefit instead.

If the employee was in fact eligible to receive a payment but too much was paid, the Social Security office need not be informed.

Where the tax year in which an overpayment was made has not ended at the time the error is discovered, the employer should reimburse the State and decide whether to make attempts to recover the overpayment from the employee. If the employee is still employed, the employer is not entitled to deduct the amount from his or her salary without his or her written consent unless of course such a deduction has already been authorised.

All such errors must be recorded in the maternity/sickness records maintained by the employer. The records must be corrected even if the employer is not successful in recovering the payment from the employee. Any money deducted from the payment or recovered must be paid back to the Inland Revenue Accounts office.

Insufficient SMP

If too little SMP has been paid to an employee and a form SMP1 has been incorrectly issued to the employee, her local Social Security office should be contacted immediately so that they can check whether a State benefit has been incorrectly paid. Arrears due and owing to the employee should be paid as soon as the error is discovered and the appropriate records should be amended, namely the current P11 and/or wage records and the employee's maternity records.

If an SMP1 has not been issued, there is no need to inform the local Social Security office. Instead the employer should simply pay the arrears owing to the employee and record them as normal on the current P11 and/or wage records and maternity records.

SMP Mistake in the Current Tax Year Records

If it comes to the employer's attention that the incorrect amount has been recorded on the P11, the incorrect figure should be crossed out (but it should remain readable) and the correct figure inserted.

If the employer has recovered too much or not enough from the NIC payments, the next monthly payment should be adjusted or instead the amount should be corrected in the payment of any end-of-year balance due.

SMP Mistake in the Previous Tax Years Records

If the mistake is discovered after the end-of-year tax returns have been sent to the Inland Revenue Accounts office, the employer should try to ascertain whether the Accounts office still holds them or whether they have been sent to the Central Office in Newcastle. If the Accounts office still holds them, then they may be adjusted accordingly. If, however, they have already been sent to the Central Office in

Newcastle, the employer should contact the local Social Security office for advice. The employer must not correct the records without first seeking advice. A six year time limit exists for adjustments.

Records

Statutory Records

Every employer is obliged to maintain certain specified records in respect of employees who have ben absent from work due to pregnancy and who have received SMP. These records are to be maintained for a period of three years after the end of the tax year in which the MPP ends.

For each relevant employee, the records must record the timing and payment of SMP. The records must include the following information.

- The date of the first day of absence from work wholly or partly because of pregnancy or confinement as notified by the employee and, if different, the date of the first day when such absence commenced.
- The weeks in that tax year in which SMP was paid and the amount paid in each week.
- Any week in that tax year which was within the employee's MPP but for which no payment of SMP was made and the reasons no payment was made.

The employer must also retain for three years after the end of the tax year in which the MPP ends, the original medical certificate or other evidence which the employee has given to the employer relating to the EWC. This could include the actual date of the birth if that is the evidence which the employee provided to the employer as evidence of confinement. The employer shall not, therefore, retain a birth certificate since a record of the date of the birth will suffice.

A copy of the certificate or other such evidence as provided by the employee will suffice where an employer has had to return the original to the employee in order for her to be able to make a claim for a State benefit.

Accounting Records

There is a requirement for employers to maintain proper accounting records for the purposes of reclaiming SMP and NIC compensation from the Inland Revenue. The records which must be kept are as follows.

- The SMP payments on the official Deductions Working Sheet (Form P11). The full amount of NIC due must also be recorded.

- The total SMP payments for the year of the official End of Year Return form (Form P14). The full amount of NIC due must also be recorded.

Both of these forms are supplied by the Inland Revenue Accounts office.

- The total gross SMP and SSP payment and the total amount of NIC compensation on the employer's annual statement, declaration and certificate (P35).

Additional Records

In addition to the records mentioned above which an employer is obliged to keep, there are a number of other records which an employer may find useful to maintain.

In relation to maternity the DSS have suggested that the following records may prove useful for an employer.

- Details of in-house notification rules for maternity absence and the dates on which relevant employees give their notice. These records would prove to be useful to an employer where he or she has decided that the employee is not eligible to receive SMP because notification was given late but where the employee disagrees with that decision.

- Copies of current applications for formal decisions of an appeal to an Adjudication Officer, tribunal or Commissioner. Such a record could prove useful for an employer awaiting a formal decision and to explain why payment has not as yet been made. In addition, a copy of each decision.

- The calculations of higher rate SMP in respect of each employee and the calculation of the eight week average earnings.

A DSS inspector has the authority to enter the employer's offices at any reasonable time in order to inspect the records. Penalties are incurred if an employer does not comply with an inspector's reasonable request.

Non-compliance with the requirement to keep the necessary records is a criminal offence. The offence is punishable by a fine of up to £400 per offence. The continued failure following conviction is punishable by a further fine for each day of the continued failure.

Insolvency of Employer

If an employer becomes insolvent, liability for payment of SMP passes from the employer to the Secretary of State. This happens from the week in which the employer first became insolvent until the end of the MPP.

Checklist: Where SMP is not payable

An employee is not entitled to payments of SMP in the following situations.

- If she is not employed into the QW.
- If she has not been continuously employed for at least 26 weeks into the QW.
- If late notice or no notice is given of an intention to take maternity leave.
- If no medical evidence is provided (within a reasonable period of time).
- If she goes outside the EEA.
- If she is taken into legal custody.
- If she commences work for another employer after her confinement.

The first payment will be made as soon as practicable after the liability passes to the Secretary of State. Payments thereafter are made at weekly intervals.

Any outstanding payments which become due prior to the employer's insolvency will neverthelss remain the employer's responsibility.

Different Types of Pregnancy

Miscarriages and Stillbirths

As discussed earlier, for an employee to be eligible to receive SMP, she must be pregnant and have reached, or have been confined before reaching, the 11th week before the EWC or have given birth to a live child before that date.

"Confinement" in this context means labour resulting in the birth of a living child or the birth of a child whether living or dead after 24 weeks of pregnancy, and "confined" is therefore construed accordingly.

A woman who suffers a miscarriage before the end of the 24th week of pregnancy and is absent from work will not be absent because of confinement and therefore SMP will not be payable. If, however, a stillbirth occurs after that time (ie after the beginning of the 16th week before the EWC) SMP will still be payable.

Twins/Multiple Birth

A woman is only entitled to one SMP payment regardless of the number of children born. However, to assist her, she is entitled to a Child Allowance for each child.

Premature Birth before QW

The QW is the 15th week before the EWC. If the birth occurs before the 15th week before the EWC, an employee is still entitled to her SMP.

There are different SMP conditions in such a situation as follows:

- if the employee would but for her confinement have been in employment for a continuous period of at least 26 weeks ending with the week immediately preceding the 14th week before the EWC, and

- her normal weekly earnings for the period of eight weeks ending with the week immediately preceding the week of her confinement are not less than the lower earnings limit in force immediately before the commencement of the week of her confinement.

In addition, the employee must, if reasonably practicable give notice of the date when the baby was born within 21 days of the birth.

Birth before the EWC

So long as the birth is after the commencement of the MPP, an employee's entitlement to SMP is not affected if the birth is earlier than the EWC.

Premature Birth after the QW but before MPP

An employee's entitlement to SMP is not affected by a birth before the MPP but after the QW. The only effect will be that the MPP will start to run from the week after the week in which the birth took place. Any employee is obliged if reasonably practicable to give notice of the date of the birth within 21 days of the event.

Contractual Maternity Pay

An employer may make provision in the employee's contract of employment for her to receive maternity pay for periods in excess of SMP as part of her contract. This contractual payment may or may not be in addition to SMP or Maternity Allowance (MA). The employer may recover the SMP element *only* from the Government.

Questions and Answers

Q: What should I do if I realise that an error has been made and an SMP1 has been issued by mistake?

A: *The employee should be told immediately that an error has been made and her DSS office should be informed in order to avoid the payment of state benefit in error. Then SMP should be paid.*

Q: What should I do if I discover that SMP has been paid when it should not have been?

A: *The DSS should be notified and advised of the employee's details and the date of the period concerned. The employee will have to complete the appropriate form entitling her to claim state benefit. If you discover that the SMP has been paid at too high a rate, you do not need to notify the employee's DSS office. Instead, you should correct the mistake in the maternity and wages records and any money that has been wrongly deducted or recovered should be paid back to the Inland Revenue. You may wish to attempt to recover the overpayment from the employee concerned but in any event your records must be adjusted even if no recovery is made.*

Q: Am I obliged to keep any records of maternity pay?

A: *Yes. You are obliged to maintain certain records for three years after the end of the tax year to which the records relate. Details which must be recorded are as follows:*

- *the weeks for which SMP was paid*
- *the amount of SMP paid in each week*
- *the dates of any weeks within the MPP for which SMP was not paid and the reasons for the non-payment*
- *maternity certificates (MATB1) given by employees in receipt of SMP*

> - *copies of any MATB1 forms where the employer has returned the original to the employee due to the employer's liability to pay SMP ending.*
>
> *Failure to keep the appropriate records is a criminal offence punishable by a fine not exceeding £400 per offence. Continued failure following conviction is punishable by a further fine up to £40.00 per day for each day of the continued failure.*
>
> *Employers are also obliged to maintain proper accounting records in order to reclaim SMP or NIC compensation from the Inland Revenue:*
>
> - *record SMP payments on the employee's Deduction Working Sheets (P11)*
> - *record the total SMP payments on the employer's End of Year Returns (P14)*
> - *record on your Annual Statement, Declaration and Certificate (P35) the total gross SMP payments and the total sum of NIC compensation on the SMP.*

Q: If an employee works for only one day during a week, how much SMP would she lose as a result?

A: *She would lose a full week's SMP entitlement. SMP is always counted in terms of full weeks commencing on a Sunday and so it makes no difference if an employee works for only one day of a week or six days of a week since that week's entitlement will automatically be lost.*

Q: To what extent would I be responsible for making maternity payments to an eligible employee?

A: *If an employee is not eligible to receive SMP, Maternity Allowance is available to her if she has been employed or self-employed and has paid standard rate NIC for the relevant period as detailed earlier. Maternity allowance is paid by Social Security the Department of and not the employer. However, SMP is primarily the responsibility of the employer.*

Q: Does a written contract of employment need to exist for an employee to be entitled to an SMP payment?

A: *No.*

Q: Can I pay more than the minimum SMP entitlement?

A: *Yes, provision can be made in the employee's contract of employment for her to receive maternity pay in excess of the statutory minimum.*

Q: Can I make deductions from any SMP payments?

A: *Yes, in effect SMP is to be treated in the same way as an employee's normal earnings since it is subject to both PAYE and NIC and so any deductions which an employer is entitled to make from an employee's wages can also be made from payments of SMP.*

Q: What should I do if I decide that an employee is not eligible to receive SMP?

A: *If the employee has worked for you in the QW you are obliged to complete form SMP1 within seven days of making the decision that she is not entitled to SMP. You must also return to her any maternity certificate which she may have given to you. She would then be in a position to apply for MA.*

Q: What happens if I become insolvent and am therefore unable to make the appropriate payments of SMP to an eligible employee?

A: *If an employer is insolvent then outstanding payments of SMP from the week of the insolvency become the responsibility of the Secretary of State. However, any outstanding payments which became due prior to the insolvency remain your responsibility.*

Q: What should I do if the employee gives me less than 21 days' notice of her absence?

A: *You should consider the employee's circumstances and if you feel she had a good reason for not complying with the time limit, then you should accept it. If you do not accept the reason as a sufficiently good one then the employee can request a written statement from you. If she is not satisfied with your reason she can apply for a formal decision of an Adjudication Officer.*

Q: Is SMP payable for 18 weeks regardless of whether the woman is on short-term or long-term maternity leave?

A: *No. When the woman resumes work after the 14 weeks leave, her entitlement to SMP ceases.*

Q: Can an employee receive SMP and Statutory Sick Pay (SSP) at the same time?

A: *No. There is a strict provision that an employee cannot receive SMP and SSP at the same time. Consequently, once the MPP has begun, the employee is disqualified from receiving SSP until the MPP has ended.*

6 Disputes and Appeals

If an employer refuses to pay an employee SMP or fails to pay the amount which the employee is entitled to receive, the employee has the right to challenge the employer's decision.

Internal Grievance Procedure

It is usually advisable for an employee firstly to address the dispute through the available internal grievance procedure since the dispute may well be resolved at this stage without the need to apply to an Adjudication Officer. In any event, even if the internal grievance process proves to be unsuccessful, the employee will have had an opportunity to prepare her case which can now be presented to an Adjudication Officer.

A Written Statement

If an employer decides not to pay the employee SMP or pays her less than the employee thinks she is entitled to receive, the employee may request the employer to provide an explanation of his or her decision. However, if the employee is not satisfied with the reason provided by the employer, the employee has the right to ask the employer to provide her with a written statement.

The written statement should address the following matters:

- the weeks in the maternity absence which the employer regards as weeks for which SMP is payable, and
- how much SMP the employer considers the employee is entitled to for each of these weeks, and
- the reason(s) the employer does not regard himself or herself as liable to pay SMP for other weeks.

Where the employer decides that he or she has no liability to make payments of SMP to the employee, the employer's obligation to provide the employee with details as mentioned above is to do so "within seven days of the decision being made, or, if earlier, within 21 days of the day the woman gave notice of her intended absence or of her confinement if that had occurred".

Application to an Adjudication Officer

If the employee is not satisfied with her employer's decision not to pay her SMP or SSP, then she can ask the Adjudication Officer for a formal decision.

Who is the Adjudication Officer?

The Adjudication Officer is a Social Security officer appointed by the Secretary of State who is responsible for making independent decisions on disputes in respect of SMP, SSP and other Social Security benefits. The Adjudication Officer is the first of the adjudicating authorities to look at disputes in relation to such matters. Despite working from DSS offices, they are nevertheless independent of the DSS.

Who Can Apply for a Decision?

Only the employee or an officer of the DSS can apply for a decision from an Adjudication Officer. The employer obviously does not have the right; he or she has to make up his or her own mind as to the liability to pay SMP, SSP and other such benefits. However, the employer does have the right to appeal against the Adjudication Officer's decision.

Before an employee applies for a formal decision from an Adjudication Officer, an employee is expected to have already asked the employer to provide her with a written statement.

Time Limits

In the case of SMP, the employee must apply within six months of the earliest day on which a dispute over SMP liability arose.

Procedure

The application must be in writing and in the case of an SMP dispute, the form SMP14 should be used. The application should specify the grounds on which the employer has relied in refusing to make the appropriate payments and the period for which this refusal has lasted. Therefore, neither party will actually appear in person before the Adjudication Officer. If the Adjudication Officer should require any further evidence or information from the employee in respect of the matter prior to making a decision the Adjudication Officer will ask the appropriate Social Security official to assist in providing it.

The Powers of the Adjudication Officer

An Adjudication Officer has the ability to do the following.

- Refer the dispute to the Secretary of State in certain situations. The disputes which are seen to justify a referral to the Secretary of State are decisions which involve the following questions:
  - whether an individual is, or was, an employer or employee of another
  - whether an employee's employment was continuous
  - the amount that is to be paid or alternatively deducted
  - whether two or more contracts or two or more employers should be treated as one for the purposes of SMP
  - whether an employer can receive NIC compensation on SMP paid.
- Reach a decision about the dispute.
- Refer the claim to a Social Security Appeal Tribunal.

A formal decision will be sent by the Adjudication Officer to both parties concerned and if the Adjudication Officer overturns the employer's decision not to make payments to the employee, then the appropriate payments must be paid within the fixed period unless, of course, the employer decides to appeal the Adjudication Officer's decision.

Appeal Against an Adjudication Officer's Decision

Both the employer and the employee have the right to appeal against a formal decision of the Adjudication Officer. Full details of this right will be included in the formal decision which will, of course, have been sent to both parties.

Time Limit

There is a three month time limit from the date when the claimant received notice of the Adjudication Officer's decision. It is a strict time limit and an applicant can only lodge an appeal outside this time limit if the applicant can establish that there were "special reasons" for the delay.

Notice

Notification of the hearing date will be sent to the parties concerned at least 10 clear days before the hearing date. In addition, prior to the hearing, each party will receive the other party's evidence and a copy of all the papers which the Adjudication Officer proposes to put before the tribunal at the hearing. This will include the Adjudication Officer's statement dealing with the facts and the law of the case in dispute.

The Hearing

The tribunal hearing the appeal consists of a Chairman and two lay members. The Chairman is a senior lawyer. The Chairman must make an accurate record of the proceedings and the tribunal's decision. The hearing will be an oral hearing and will be held in public unless the appellant specifically requests the hearing to be held in private, or if the tribunal takes the view that it would be more appropriate to be held in private due, for example, to the particularly private nature of the hearing.

The hearing is intended to be as informal as possible.

The parties can be represented or can act in person. Each party will be invited by the tribunal to state his or her case. The decision will always be provided in writing and a copy will be provided for the parties as soon as possible following the hearing.

Further Appeal

There is a further right of appeal following the tribunal's decision to a Social Security Commissioner provided leave is granted by the Chairman or a Commissioner. In addition, further appeal can also be made to the Court of Appeal if there is a significant point of law in issue.

Appeal to a Social Security Commissioner

An Appeal to the Commissioner against a tribunal's decision can only be made on a point of law and with the permission of the Chairman or a Commissioner.

Who is a Social Security Commissioner?

Social Security Commissioners are appointed by the Crown and must be lawyers of at least 10 years' standing.

Who May Appeal

Only the categories of persons detailed below are entitled to appeal against a tribunal's decision.

- The employee.
- The employer.
- The Adjudication Officer.
- A Trade Union or any other such association existing to promote the interests and welfare of its members. This is on the proviso that the employee at the time of the appeal is a member and was so immediately before the question in dispute arose or the question is one concerning the entitlement of a deceased member.
- An association of employers of which the employer is a member at the time of the appeal and of which he or she was also a member immediately prior to the question now in dispute.

Procedure

If the Chairman of the Social Security Appeal Tribunal does not allow leave to appeal, a party has 42 days in which to apply direct to the Social Security Commissioner for leave to appeal.

If the Chairman of the Social Security Appeal Tribunal grants the party leave to appeal, then the appeal documentation must be lodged, together with a copy of the original tribunal's decision and a copy of the Chairman's decision granting leave for the appeal within 42 days.

The party lodging the appeal will receive an acknowledgement and the other party will be sent a copy of the Notice of Appeal. The Respondent is entitled to send his or her written observations on the appeal to the Commissioner within 30 days of having received the Notice of Appeal. Thereafter, additional written observations may be submitted by either party in reply within 30 days.

The party lodging the appeal will receive an acknowledgement and the other party will be sent a copy of the Notice of Appeal. The Respondent is entitled to send his or her written observations on the Appeal to the Commissioner within 30 days of having received the Notice of Appeal.

Thereafter, additional written observations may be submitted by either party in reply within 30 days.

Hearing

The appeal would usually be heard by a single Commissioner, although if the appeal involves a particularly complex area of law, then three Commissioners may be required to hear the dispute. The appeal is generally decided on the basis of the case papers although, should one of the parties or the Commissioner take the view that the matter cannot be properly decided without conducting an oral hearing, then an oral hearing will be duly held.

Appeal to the Court of Appeal/Court of Session

As mentioned earlier, there is a further right of appeal on a point of law to the Court of Appeal or the Court of Session in Scotland. Permission for a further appeal must first be sought from a Commissioner or if the Commissioner refuses to grant leave for the further appeal then leave can be sought from the Court of Appeal itself. An application for leave further to appeal must be made within three months of the date on which the applicant received written notification of the decision being appealed.

Disputes Reserved for the Secretary of State

As mentioned and detailed earlier, some disputes are reserved for the Secretary of State to deal with.

Procedure

The applicant must send an application in the format approved by the Secretary of State. The Secretary will then either make a decision on the dispute or alternatively appoint an official to hold a suitable inquiry to assist the Secretary prior to the decision being made. If the circumstances are such that the Secretary requires an inquiry to be conducted prior to making his or her decision, then the appointed official in charge of the inquiry can request individuals to attend in order to give evidence or produce documentation.

If the Secretary of State requires further information from either party and the parties fail to provide the information requested within 10 days following a written request, the party resisting is guilty of committing a criminal offence. The offence is punishable by a fine of up to £400 and subsequent to a conviction, a further £40 fine per day thereafter should the information still not be forthcoming.

The decision reached by the Secretary of State will be given to the applicant in writing. The written decision will also inform the parties of their right to request further details.

Review

If new facts subsequently come to the attention of the Secretary and he or she takes the view that the earlier decision had been given on the basis of a mistake or ignorance of a material fact or simply misapplication of the law, then the Secretary may decide to review the earlier decision.

Appeal

Decisions of the Secretary of State are binding on Adjudication Officers, Social Security Appeal Tribunals and Social Security Commissioners. An appeal can therefore only be made on a point of law and the appeal can only be conducted by the High Court or the Court of Session.

Judicial Review

If a party concerned is aggrieved by the decision of the Secretary of State then it may be challenged by submitting an application for a judicial review of the decision. Such an application for a judicial review is usually submitted within three months.

Review as Opposed to Appeal

As an alternative to lodging an appeal against the decision of an Adjudication Officer an application may be made for the decision simply to be reviewed. The review will usually be conducted by an Adjudication Officer although he or she may refer the matter to a tribunal. The Adjudication Officer can review his or her decision if:

- the decision was made without being aware of all of the material facts, or
- there was a mistake as to the facts, or
- there was a misapplication of law, or
- circumstances have changed since the decision was made, or
- the decision was based on a question which was not decided by an Adjudication Officer and that decision has subsequently been reviewed.

A review can be requested at any time by writing to the

local Social Security office which forwarded the notice of the decision which is now being challenged. The application should clearly set out the reasons for requesting the review.

The review should be conducted within 14 days of the application if possible.

The Adjudication Officer has a number of options available to him or her in conducting the review. He or she can:

- refuse to review the decision, or
- review the decision but decline to alter it, or
- review the decision and alter it, or
- refer the matter to the appropriate regional tribunal.

If the decision is reviewed, the Adjudication Officer will again issue a formal decision. There are the same rights of appeal against this reviewed decision as there are with an initial decision should a party remain dissatisfied with the decision.

Enforcement of Formal Decisions

If a formal decision is issued and the employee is entitled to a certain amount of SMP from her employer, there is a strict timetable within which the employer must comply with the decision and pay the employee the amount to which she is entitled.

Time Limit

The employer is obliged to pay the appropriate amount on the first "payday" after the time limit for all possible appeals has expired or leave to appeal has been refused. If the appropriate amount has not been paid by the employer and the time limit for appealing against the formal decision has lapsed and no other appeal has been lodged in respect of that decision, the Secretary of State will automatically assume liability for the payment of the sum due.

"Payday" has been defined in the legislation as follows:

"a day on which it has been agreed, or it is the normal practice between an employer or former employer and a woman who is or was an employee, that payments by way of remuneration are to be made, or, where there is no such agreement or normal practice, the last day of a calendar month."

The timetable within which the employer must pay the appropriate amount is not later than the first payday after:

(a) where an appeal has been brought, the day on which the employer or former employer receives notification that it has been finally disposed of

(b) where leave to appeal has been refused and there remains no further opportunity to apply for leave, the day on which the employer or former employer receives notification of the refusal, and

(c) in any other case, the day on which the time for bringing an appeal expires.

However, there are two exceptions identified which are as follows.

- Where it is impractical, due to the employer's or former employer's accounting methods for payment to be made on the first payday then payment shall "be met not later than the next following payday".

- Where the employer or former employer would not have normally paid the employee for her work in the week in question as early as the payday, then the payment "shall be met on the first day on which the woman would have been remunerated for her work in that week".

Failure to Comply with the Timetable for Payment

If the employer fails to make payment in accordance with the timetable outlined, then, as mentioned above, liability to make those payments shall be that of the Secretary of State and not the employer. Therefore, the employee can recover the appropriate sum directly from the Secretary of State.

The Secretary of State can as a result bring charges against the employer for his or her failure to make the appropriate payments following the decision that such payments should be made.

In addition, it is a criminal offence for the employer not to comply with the decision and the offence is punishable by a fine. A person shall be the subject of a penalty where there is contravention "without reasonable excuse". Therefore, for failure to pay SMP within the time limits, there is a maximum fine of £400 for any one offence.

Questions and Answers

Q: What should I do if I decide that SMP is not payable to an employee?

A: *The employee should be informed of the position and may request a written statement from you setting out the reasons for the decision.*

Q: Can the employee take any action against me for my refusal to make SMP payments?

A: *Yes, an employee who remains dissatisfied with the reasons given by the employer in the written statement, may ask an Adjudication Officer for a formal decision.*

Q: If the employee decides to request a formal decision from an Adjudication Officer would I have to appear before him or her to put my case?

A: *No, both you and the employee will simply be asked to put your observations in writing together with any supporting evidence.*

Q: If it transpires that my decision was incorrect and the benefits should in fact have been paid to the employee, will I incur any fine/penalty for the error?

A: *Not initially. However, there is a strict timetable for payment of the amount due and owing (namely the first payday after the time limits for all possible appeals has expired or leave to appeal has been refused). If you do not comply with the time limits, the Secretary of State will assume liability for payment and he or she will then have the right to bring charges against you for your failure to pay. The fine will not exceed £400 for any one offence. However, continued failure to pay after a conviction will result in a further fine of up to £20 per day until payment.*

7 Health and Safety

The EC Pregnant Workers Directive includes a number of measures to provide protection for the health and safety at work of those workers who are pregnant, those who have recently given birth and those who are breast-feeding. The Directive itself is only directly enforceable against state employers and not private sector employers. Some of it's provisions have been implemented in TURERA 1993 and others will be implemented by way of statutory instrument.

The underlying assumption of the Directive is that pregnant workers, or those who have recently given birth, are particularly vulnerable and face special risks to their health and safety and for this reason are entitled to additional protection.

EC Pregnant Workers Directive

To Whom does the Directive Apply?

The Directive applies to three categories of workers:

(a) pregnant workers
(b) workers who have recently given birth
(c) workers who are breast-feeding.

These categories have been specifically defined in Article 2 of the Directive as follows.

- **Pregnant worker.**
  "A pregnant worker who informs her employer of her condition, in accordance with national legislation and/or national practice."

- **Worker who has recently given birth.**
  "A worker who has recently given birth within the meaning of national legislation and/or national practice and who informs her employer of her condition, in accordance with that legislation and/or practice."

- **Worker who is breast-feeding.**
  "A worker who is breast-feeding within the meaning of national legislation and/or national practice and who informs her employer of her condition in accordance with that legislation and/or practice."

It is clear from the above definitions that to fall within the provisions of the Directive, a worker must actually have informed her employer that she is either pregnant, has recently given birth or is breast-feeding.

Requirements under the Directive

Once the worker has informed her employer of her condition, the employer is thereafter required to take the measures detailed in the Directive in order to safeguard her health and safety. The measures to be taken are as follows.

- **Assessment (Article 4)**
  Employers are obliged to carry out an assessment of the worker's working conditions in order to ascertain whether there is any potential risk to her health and safety which may affect her pregnancy.

  The employer is obliged to assess the physical, biological and chemical hazards in the worker's workplace which may create potential risks.

  Article 4 of the Directive specifically states that assessment should take place in respect of "all activities liable to involve a specific risk of exposure to the agents, processes or working conditions". Annex I of the Directive provides a non-exhaustive list of the "agents, processes and working conditions" referred to above. The list is divided into three categories — physical agents, biological agents and chemical agents (see Figure 7).

The actual risk to the worker depends on the "nature, degree and duration of the exposure" in each particular case. Therefore, each case has to be looked at on its own merits.

Once the assessment has taken place, the employer must decide what appropriate measures to take in response to the results of the assessment.

The results of the assessment and the measures which the employer has decided to take must be communicated to the worker and/or her representative.

Figure 7: Annex I of the Directive

Physical Agents

Those agents which are regarded as agents causing foetal lesions and/or likely to disrupt placental attachment, particularly shocks, vibration or movement; the handling of loads entailing risks; risks; noise; ionising radiation; non-ionising radiation; extremes of cold or heat; movements and postures, travelling and mental and physical fatigue and other physical burdens.

Biological Agents

Agents of risks groups 2, 3 and 4 within the meaning of Article 2(d) nos. 2, 3 and 4 of Directive 90/679 EEC insofar as it is known that the agents or the therapeutic measures necessitated by the agents endanger the health of pregnant women and the foetus.

Chemical Agents

Substances labelled R40, R45, R46 and R47 under Directive 67/548/EEC; chemical agents in Annex I to Directive 90/394/EEC; mercury and mercury derivatives; antimitotic drugs; carbon monoxide; chemical agents of known and dangerous percutaneous absorption insofar as the above are known to endanger the health of pregnant women and the unborn child.

- **Adjustment of Working Conditions (Article 5)**

   Where the assessment reveals a risk to the health and safety of the worker, the employer must make a temporary adjustment to her working conditions and/or her hours of work so that she is not exposed to the risk.

   However, if having ascertained that there is a risk, it is in fact not "technically and/or objectively feasible or cannot reasonably be required on duly substantiated grounds" the employee should be moved to another job to avoid exposure to the risk.

   In the event that the placing of the worker on an alternative job is also not "technically and/or objectively feasible and cannot reasonably be required on duly substantiated grounds", the employee is to be given leave for such period as is necessary for her health and safety. During any such period of absence, the worker's contractual rights subsist.

- **Specific Risks (Article 6)**

   In addition to the list of agents, processes and working conditions outlined in Annex I and detailed in Figure 7, Annex II of the Directive provides a non-exhaustive list of "specific risks" which are harmful to two of the categories of relevant workers outlined earlier, namely the pregnant worker and the breast-feeding worker. The substances outlined in Annex II are such that a worker who is either pregnant or breast-feeding should not be exposed to them (see Figure 8).

- **Night Work (Article 7)**

   The three categories of workers defined earlier must not be obliged to perform night work during their pregnancy and for a certain period of time after the birth. The period of time after the birth during which a worker is not obliged to undertake night work is to be determined by the national authority competent for health and safety.

Figure 8: Annex II of the Directive

Pregnant Workers

Physical Agents

Work in hyperbaric atmosphere, for example, pressurised enclosures and underwater diving.

Biological Agents

Toxoplasma, rubella virus (unless the pregnant worker is proved to be adequately immunised).

Chemical Agents

Lead and lead derivatives capable of being absorbed by the human organism.

Breast-feeding Workers

Working Conditions

Underground mining work.

Chemical Agents

Lead and lead derivatives capable of being absorbed by the human organism.

However, the obligation not to engage in night work is only effective if the worker submits a medical certificate stating that night work should not be undertaken for health and safety reasons. If such a medical certificate is submitted, an employer should, for example, transfer the worker concerned to daytime work for the requisite period. However, there is a proviso in Article 7 stating that if a transfer is "not technically and/or objectively feasible or cannot reasonably be required on duly substantiated grounds", then the employer may give the worker leave or an extension of her maternity leave.

Checklist: Pregnant Workers Directive

- Employer is informed by employee that she is either pregnant, has recently given birth or is breast-feeding.

- Employer has to assess the nature, degree and duration of exposure to risk.

- Decides what appropriate measures to take to avoid exposure.

- Reports to the worker the result of the assessment and the measures to be taken.

- Implements those measures.

- Temporarily adjusts the employee's working conditions.

- Night work — employee must provide a medical certificate.

- Workers should continue working with VDUs but research is continuing in this area.

TURERA 1993 Provisions

TURERA 1993 will introduce a new right for pregnant women who are unable to continue working for health and safety reasons. The new provisions come into force in October 1994. Previously an employee could fairly dismiss in such circumstances. This will no longer be the case. Section 22 will confer new rights on women to be suspended from work on grounds of maternity. These rights are set out in detail in Sch.3 to the Act.

An employee who is pregnant, or has recently given birth or is breast-feeding (as defined above) is to be treated as suspended on maternity grounds if it would be in contravention of any enactment or any recommendation in the code of practice issued under s.16 of the Health and Safety at Work Act 1974 for her to continue to work. An employee is regarded as suspended "so long as, she continues to be employed by her employer but is not provided with work or does not perform the work she normally performed before suspension."

However, s.46(1) provides that where "an employer has available suitable alternative work for an employee the employee has the right to be offered to be provided with it before being suspended on maternity grounds."

Alternative Work

The alternative available work must be of a nature which is suitable to the employee and appropriate for her to undertake in her condition as an employee who is pregnant, has recently given birth or is breast-feeding. It is expressly provided that if the terms and conditions of the alternative work differ from those applicable to the job the employee normally performs, then they must not be "substantially less favourable".

Failure to be Offered Available Suitable Alternative Work

An employee has the right to bring a complaint to an industrial tribunal if her employer has failed to offer her such alternative work. The complaint must be lodged with the tribunal within three months of the first day of suspension (s.46(3)). If the employee is successful and the tribunal makes a finding in her favour, the tribunal may make an award of compensation against the employer of an amount such as the tribunal considers just and equitable taking into account:

- the employer's failure to offer the alternative work, and

- the loss sustained by the employee which is attributable to the employer's failure.

Remuneration whilst Suspended

Section 47(1) provides that an employee who is suspended on maternity grounds is entitled to be paid her normal weekly remuneration whilst she is suspended. The section does not, however, make any reference to her entitlement to non-cash benefits although since this section is seeking to implement the Directive, it would seem that non-cash benefits should continue during the period of suspension.

This remuneration is subject to her not having unreasonably refused to accept an offer of suitable alternative work during the relevant period. If the employee does unreasonably refuse such an offer, she will forfeit the right to be paid during any period of suspension.

Remedy

If the employer fails to make payment in whole or in part to the employee, she may present a complaint to an industrial tribunal on the basis that her employer has failed to pay the whole or any part of her remuneration to which she is entitled. The remuneration which the employee receives goes towards discharging the employer's liability under these provisions. If a finding is made in favour of the employee, the tribunal may order the employer to pay outstanding remuneration owed to the employee.

The complaint must be lodged within three months beginning with the first day payment is not made, or within such further period if the tribunal considers that it was not reasonably practicable for her to comply with the three month time limit.

Implementing Regulations

A consultative document has been issued by the Health and Safety Commission (HSC) with a view to implementing the remaining provisions of the EC Directive on pregnant workers.

In line with its strategy of keeping requirements as simple and rationalised as possible, the HSC proposes that

> ### Checklist: Suitable Alternative Work
>
> - If there is any available suitable alternative work it should be offered to the employee.
> - The employee could lodge a complaint with an industrial tribunal if available suitable alternative work is not offered to her.
> - If there is no suitable alternative work available the employee, whilst temporarily suspended, is entitled to receive remuneration.

the health and safety provisions of the Directive should be implemented by an amendment to the Management of Health and Safety at Work Regulations. These regulations already require employers to:

- assess the risks to health and safety of their employees to which they are exposed whilst they are at work (Regulation 3) and make it clear that the assessment must have regard to groups especially at risk
- give employees information about the risks to their health and safety identified by the assessment (Regulation 8).

The Commission are proposing that the existing duty to carry out risk assessment should cover the particular risks run by those who are pregnant, those who are breast-feeding or have recently given birth and that each of these three groups should be informed of the results of the assessment.

If the results of the assessment reveal a risk to the safety or health of a new or expectant mother, employers should refer to any legislation that cover the particular risk and take corrective action. If a risk remains which would jeopardise the worker's safety or health and which is related to pregnancy or breast-feeding, the employer must follow the steps set out in Regulation 13A(2) and (3), ie change the worker's working conditions or hours of work to avoid the risk, or if that is not reasonable suspend her from work (ie give her paid leave). However, as pointed out above, s.46 of the Employment Protection (Consolidation) Act 1978 gives women the right, in these circumstances, to be offered suitable alternative employment and the right to paid leave will be lost if the employee turned down an offer of suitable alternative employment.

As regards Article 7 of the Directive (night work) Regulation 13B already requires action of an employer if a new or expectant mother has a medical certificate stating that for health and safety reasons she should not perform night work. Such employees have the right to transfer to daytime work under s.46, or if that is not possible, the employer must offer the employee paid leave from work.

Finally, Article 8 provides a minimum of two weeks paid maternity leave immediately before or immediately after the birth. The HSC does not consider that the two weeks compulsory maternity leave is an occupational health and safety matter and the Government is expected to introduce separate legislation to implement this recommendation.

Display Screen Equipment

There has been much debate about the effect visual display units (VDUs) have on women and their reproductive health. The concerns have arisen as a result of a number of reports concerning the higher levels of miscarriages and birth defects in workers working with VDUs. However, the draft guidance on the Health and Safety (Display Screen Equipment) Regulations states that as a whole the scientific studies which have been carried out in this area do "not show any link between miscarriages or birth defects and working with VDUs". As a result, the guidance specifically states that "women do not need to stop work with VDUs". However, workers who are anxious about the situation should consult their doctors or someone adequately informed in this area to give advice and information.

Further research and reviews of current scientific evidence is being undertaken in this area.

Questions and Answers

Q: What are my obligations currently if there is a maternity-related health and safety risk with one of my employees?

A: *You should use all endeavours to eliminate the risk so that her employment can continue. However, if it is not possible to eliminate sufficiently the risk, there is no statutory obligation to find her an alternative job. However, in the eventuality of dismissing her an employer should be aware that the employee could potentially bring a claim under the Sex Discrimination Act 1975. Employers would therefore be advised to be careful and consider temporary suspension.*

Q: What is the position under TURERA 1993?

A: *Section 25 with Schedule 3 provides that an employee must be offered available suitable alternative work on terms and conditions not substantially less favourable than those pertaining to her current position. If there is no available suitable alternative work then she must receive her normal remuneration during her period of suspension.*

Q: What is the position as regards pay if I have to give the worker time off since I am unable to temporarily adjust her working conditions or find her another job?

A: *The Commission had originally proposed that a worker should continue to receive her full salary or equivalent benefit. However, this was rejected by the Council of Ministers and it was instead provided that pay in such circumstances will be governed by national law.*

Q: What do I do if a worker objects to using her VDU?

A: *You should tell her that there is no evidence of a direct link between reproductive problems and VDUs and that she should continue using it. You should tell her that if she is still anxious about the situation she should discuss it with her doctor or someone else adequately informed of the current scientific information and advice in this area.*

Glossary

CHILDBIRTH
Childbirth resulting in the issue of a living child, or labour after at least 24 weeks of pregnancy resulting in the issue of a child whether alive or dead.

CORE PERIOD
The period of 13 weeks commencing six weeks before the EWC.

EUROPEAN COMMUNITY
Belgium, Denmark, Germany, France, Greece, Republic of Ireland, Italy, Luxembourg, Netherlands, Spain, Portugal, United Kingdom and Gibraltar (for Social Security matters).

EXPECTED WEEK OF CHILDBIRTH (EWC)
The week in which the baby is expected to be born.

MATERNITY ALLOWANCE (MA)
Weekly benefit paid by the Social Security to pregnant women not eligible for SMP.

MATERNITY ALLOWANCE PERIOD (MAP)
The period during which MA is paid maximum is 18 weeks.

MATERNITY ALLOWANCE TEST PERIOD
The period of 66 weeks ending with the week before the week in which the baby is due.

MATERNITY PAY PERIOD (MPP)	The period during which SMP is paid for a maximum 18 weeks.
NI	National Insurance.
PIW	Period of Incapacity for Work.
QUALIFYING WEEK (QW)	The 15th week before the EWC.
SMALL EMPLOYER	An employer who pays £20,000 or less annually in gross NI contributions.
STATUTORY MATERNITY PAY (SMP)	Weekly payment made by the employer. Payable for maximum of 18 weeks. Payable at two rates, lower and higher.
WEEK	A period of seven days beginning at midnight on Saturday and ending on Sunday.

Further Information

Conferences and Training

Attending a seminar is one of the best ways of keeping up with rapidly changing legislation, trends and new ideas. Croner Conferences and Training have 10 years' experience of running an extensive range of courses, from three-day residential to one-day seminars, all led by authoritative and experienced speakers. Courses are regularly offered on the following subjects:

Drafting Contracts of Employment
The Effective Personnel Assistant
Advanced Employment Law
Psychometric Tests: Their Selection and Use
Managing Absenteeism
Managing Sickness Absence
Going to Tribunal
Fleet Management
Payroll Management
Statutory Sick Pay
SMP and other Maternity Rights
Fair Dismissal
Employment Law Update
Introduction to Pensions

For further information on any of these courses please contact Elizabeth Wolton on 081-547 3333 quoting reference ZVQZ.

Croner In-Company Training

Courses offered on:

Employment Law **Management Skills**
Health and Safety **Dangerous Substances**
Importing/Exporting **VAT and Finance**

... and many more tailored to your needs, for all levels of staff, anywhere in Europe.

Invest in your future with croner in-company training

Our package comprises:

- participative, tailored course
- no obligation preliminary meeting
- full back-up documentation
- experienced and practical trainers
- competitive price, estimated in advance
- backed by the Croner reputation

For details of value for money, affordable courses for four or more staff, tailored to your needs, ring Claire Spraggs on 081-547 3333, quoting reference ZVQZ.

Croner In-Company Training — works harder to meet your needs.

Croner Information Services

The mix and match of Croner Information Services that you just can't do without when formulating and actioning your personnel policies. The current range of our information packages includes:

Croner's Reference Book For Employers — Known as the "Personnel Managers Bible", this service covers all the legal obligations you face as an employer, in clear precise, 'jargon free' language.

Croner's Employment Law — An authoritative and comprehensive reference ser ice covering the complex area of employment law, keeping you abreast of all the legislative changes, developments in courts and the European Law, affecting the rights of individual employees.

Croner's Personnel In Practice — A detailed reference source of tried and tested practical forms and procedures together with the UK's leading employment newsletter.

Croner's Pay And Benefits Sourcebook — Essential reading for anyone involved in designing salary packages and pay policy in a company.

Croner's Personnel Assistants Handbook — Covering all the main areas of personnel including interviewing and report writing skills, employment law contracts, recruitment and selection, health and safety and much else. It is also an essential study guide for the Certificate in Personnel Practice course.

Croner's Human Resources: Management And Strategy — Management of human resources for your organisation is critical to its progress. This service provides the hard facts and expert advice you need to develop and execute an effective Human Resources strategy.

Croner's Team Leaders Briefing — A fortnightly newsletter containing articles and advice on the day-to-day problems and issues which the team leader or supervisor faces. Topics such as recruitment, appraisal interviewing, leadership skills, etc., etc.

Croner's Industrial Relations Law – An authoritative guide on all the legal provisions which regulate the relationship between employer and trade union members and trade unions.

Croner's Employment Case Law Index — Structured to keep the busy personnel professional up to date and locate relevant facts and summaries of findings for significant cases.

Croner's Employment Law Line — A telephone advisory service which is specially designed to provide guidance with your difficult and individual employment-related problems.

If you need further information or wish to make a purchase, please ring our Customer Services on 081-547 3333 (between 8.30 am and 5.00 pm weekdays) or fax on 081-547 2638. Please quote order reference ZPLG.

Could You Use Additional Copies of this Book?

Croner's Guide to Pregnancy, SMP and Maternity Rights is a pocket book designed for practical use by all those with management responsibilities. If you are a subscriber to *Croner's Reference Book for Employers* this is one of a series of books on key areas of employment.

Are there other managers in your organisation who would benefit from having a copy to hand? If so, why not give them a copy to help them consolidate their knowledge and put into practice what they have learnt.

Additional copies at a special price of £6 plus £1 p+p per copy may be ordered by telephoning our Customer Services team on 081-547 3333 quoting reference ZVQZ.

Index

absenteeism 11
ACAS conciliation officer 14
accounting records 104–105
adjudication officer 115–18, 122
    appeal against decision 92, 116, 118–21
    application 103, 116–17
    decision 103, 116–18
    eligibility for decision 116
    powers 117–18
    procedure 117
    review 122–3
    time limits 116
Advocate General 29
agency workers 85–6
aggrieved employee 115–16
allowance *see* maternity allowance
alternative employment 42, 59, 61, 70–2, 74-5, 131, 133–5
Annual Statement, Declaration and
    Certificate (P35) 105
ante-natal care 3–17
    checklist 17
    definition 3–4
    time off work 5–13, 22
        abuse 10–11
        amount 5–7
        appointment evidence 7
        contractual rights 11–12
        during working hours 6–7
        infertility treatment 14
        pay entitlement 8–10
        qualification 5
        remedies 12–14
appeals *see* disputes and appeals
appointment evidence 5, 7, 14
armed forces 88
associated employer 57, 70, 88
"authorised absence" 34, 41

benefits
    child allowance 107
    invalidity 82
    during maternity leave 35, 44
    sickness 82
    see also maternity allowance
biological agents 128–130
birth *see* expected week of confinement (EWC);
    recently given birth
breast-feeding workers 62, 127, 128, 130–3, 135
Brown v Stockton on Tees Borough Council
    [1987] IRLR 263 72
burden of proof 59, 61, 69, 72

CA *see* Court of Appeal
Castles Walker v Northern Co-operation
    Society Ltd (unreported) 56
casual workers, seasonal/regular 79, 86–7
Caussi v Hilton International IRLR 270 48
change in circumstances 95
change of employer 87–8
chemical agents 128-130
child allowance 107
code of practice 133
Community Task Force v Rimmer (1986) IRLR 203 70
"comparable man" 21–2, 25, 26, 27–8, 29, 34
compensation 104, 133
conciliation officer *see* ACAS conciliation officer
confinement 107
    see also expected week of confinement (EWC)
contractual
    maternity leave 39, 42, 47–8, 51
    maternity pay 100, 108
    payments offset 100
    rights 11–120, 34-6, 40–1, 43-4, 55
    sick pay 100
core period 81
    see also maternity leave period
Court of Appeal (CA)119, ... 120–1
    sex discrimination 26, 27
Court of Session 120–1, 122
"custom or arrangement" 86–7

death 88, 99, 119
Deduction Working Sheets (form P11) 104, 105
deductions 99
Dekker v Stichting Vormingscentrum
 Voor Jonge Volwassed (VJV-Centrum)
 Plus (1991) IRLR 27 .... 22–4, 33
  sex discrimimation 22–5, 27, 28, 75
Department of Social Security
  disputes and appeals 92, 117–20
  inspector 105
  maternity allowance (MA) 79–82
  maternity pay 105, 106
  official 116, 117, 121
  see also adjudication officer
Dhamrait v United Biscuits Ltd 8
Directives 30
  76/207/EEC 22, 27, 33
  90/394/EEC 129
  90/679/EEC 129
  92/85/EEC 79
  Article 10(2) 62
  see also Equal Treatment Directive;
    Pregnant Workers Directive
discipline 10–11
disentitlement of statutory maternity
  pay (SMP) 98–99
dismissal
  "deemed" 53
  under "indefinite contract" 29
  maternity 60–2
  after maternity leave 39–40, 42, 57, 58, 59
  reasons 21–2, 24, 25, 29, 61–2, 72–3
  for redundancy 57, 69–70, 71–2
display screen equipment 132, 136
disputes and appeals 105, 115–26
  adjudication officer 115–19
  formal decisions, enforcement of 123–5
  further appeal 119–21
  internal grievance procedure 115
  reserved for Secretary of State 121–2
  review as opposed to appeal 122–3
  written statement 115–16
domestic law 27

Dowuona v John Lewis plc (1987) ICR 788 51

early return 40
earnings
    statutory maternity pay regarded as 99
    weekly 83–4, 88–9, 95, 98
    see also lower earnings limit; payment
EAT *see* Employment Appeal Tribunal
EC *see* European Community
ECJ *see* European Court of Justice
EDC *see* expected date of confinement
Edgar v Girgione Inns Ltd, COIT 1803/13 7
Edgell v Lloyds Register of Shipping
    [1977] IRLR 463 55
employee
    definition 36
    unable/incapable of acting on own behalf 101
employer insolvency 106
employment
    interruption 52
    nature of 53–6
    place of 55, 56, 59
    suitable/appropriate 59, 61
    termination 84
    see also alternative employment; working
Employment Act 1980 3
Employment Appeal Tribunal (EAT)
    redundancy 70, 72
    return to work 46
    sex discrimination 20–1, 26, 27
Employment Protection (Consolidation) Act 1978
    ante-natal care 3–14
        abuse of right to time off 10–11
        contractual rights 11–12
        remedies 12–14
    health and safety 136
    redundancy 57, 69, 70, 71, 73–4, 75
    return to work
        dismissals 57, 60–2
        long-term maternity leave 43, 47, 53–5
        non-reinstatement 57–8, 59
        short-term maternity leave 41

Employment Protection (Employment in
    Aided Schools) Order 198 158
End of Year Returns (P14) 105
England
    courts 22
    Dekker and *Hertz* cases 27–8
    versus the European Community (EC) 22–9
        comparative approach 21–2, 25–9, 34
        uniqueness approach 20, 24, 27
EP(C)A *see* Employment Protection
    (Consolidation) Act 1978
Equal Treatment Directive 22–5, 27, 28, 33
    76/207 . . . . 22, 27
    maternity leave 33
    return to work 40, 51
European Community (EC)
    Directives *see* Directives; Equal Treatment
        Directive; Pregnant Workers Directive
    see also England v the European
        Community (EC)
European Court of Justice (ECJ)
    maternity leave 33
    sex discrimination 22–4, 27–9
EWC *see* expected week of confinement
expected date of confinement (EDC) 83, 95
expected week of confinement
    (EWC) 34, 35, 36, 37, 38, 43, 45, 94, 104
    birth before 94, 108
    maternity pay 83
    sixth week before 36, 47, 107
    11th week before 36, 37, 91, 100, 106
        maternity allowance 80, 81
        maternity pay period (MPP) 96
        return to work 44
    14th week before 34–5, 84, 95, 107
    15th week before maternity pay 80, 83–4, 107

F W Woolworths plc v Smith (1990) ICR 45 46
failure to return after 14th week 40
Flack and Others v Kodak Ltd (1986) ICR 775 86
forces *see* armed forces
Ford v Warwickshire County Council (1983) ICR 273 86

formal decisions enforcement 123–5
fraud 10–11
Fyfe v Farmer Giles Foods (Scotland) Ltd 22

giving notice 92
Gregory v Tudsbury (1982) IRLR 267 . . . . 4, 6, 8
grievance procedure, internal 115

Handels og Kontorfunktionærenes Forbund i
    Danmark v Dansk Arbejdsgiverforening
    (1991) IRLR 31 *see Hertz* case
Hayes v Malleable Working Men's Club
    (1985) IRLR 367 . . . . 21, 26
health and safety 127–37
    checklist 132
    compensation 133
    display screen equipment 132, 136
    extended maternity leave period 39
    implementing regulations 134–6
    Pregnant Workers Directive 127–32
    suspension right 59
    Trade Union Reform and Employment
        Rights Act 1993 . . . . 127, 132
Health and Safety at Work Act 1974 133
Health and Safety Commission 134–6
    assessment 135
Health and Safety (Display Screen
    Equipment) Regulations 136
hearing 118–19, 120
Hertz case 22–4, 27, 28, 75
High Court 122
higher rate statutory maternity pay
    (SMP) 79, 82, 85, 88, 95, 105, 106
Holmes v Moore Office 1984, IRLR 299 56
hourly rate, appropriate 9
House of Lords 27–9, 33, 72
HSC *see* Health and Safety Commission

imprisonment *see* legal custody
income tax 82, 99, 101
    tax year records 101, 102, 103

see also Inland Revenue; PAYE
"indefinite contract" 29, 34
infertility treatment 14
Inland Revenue 102
    Accounts Office 100, 101, 103
insolvency 106
Institute of the Motor Industry v Harvey
    [1992] IRLR 343 48
insufficient statutory maternity pay (SMP) 102
intention to return
    confirmation 48–9
    employer notification 45–6
invalidity benefit 82

James v Eastleigh Borough Council (1990) IRLR 288 27
job
    definition 55
    suitability 59, 61
John Menzies GB Ltd v Porter IRLB 457 70
judicial review 122

legal custody 96, 98–99
LEL *see* lower earnings limit
"less favourabl" 59
Llewellyn v Wigglesworth Ltd (unreported) 56
Lloyds Bank Ltd v Secretary of State
    of Employment (1979) IRLR 41 86
long-term maternity leave and return to work 42–59
    continuously employed until prior to
        11th week 34, 43, 44
    intention to return
        confirmation/notification 45–6, 48–9, 65
    nature of work 53–6
    notice before commencement 45
    notification, late 46
    place of work 55, 56, 59
    postponement by employee 50–1
    postponement by employer 52–3
    in previous capacity 55–6, 59
    qualification 43–6
    redundancy 70

```
            reinstatement ............................. 57–9
            timing of absence .......................... 47
            versus short-term ......................... 34–5
lower earnings limit (LEL) ................... 83–4, 88, 107
lower rate statutory maternity pay (SMP) ..... 79, 82, 88, 96
lump sum ................................... 100–101


MA see maternity allowance
MA1 form ......................................... 80
Management of Health and Safety
    at Work Regulations ........................... 135
MATB1 form ................................. 80, 94–5
maternity absence notification .................. 91–4, 104
            change in circumstances .................... 95
            checklist .................................. 95
            employee, aggrieved ....................... 92
            giving notice .............................. 92
            medical evidence ......................... 94–5
            notification requirements .................. 91–4
Maternity Allowance and Statutory Maternity Pay
    Regulations 1994 .............................. 79
maternity allowance (MA) ...................... 79–82
            claim ...................................... 80
            eligibility ................................. 80
            payment ............................. 79, 81–2
            test period ................................ 80
maternity allowance period (MAP) .................... 81
maternity certificate ..................... 80, 83, 94–5, 96
    see also MATB1 form
maternity dismissals .............................. 60–2
maternity leave and return to work ................ 33–67
            dismissals ............................... 60–2
            non-reinstatement other than redundancy ..... 57–9
                burden of proof ........................ 59
                small employers ..................... 57–8, 59
            suspension rights ........................ 48, 59
    see also long-term; short-term
maternity leave period (MLP) .................. 35, 36–42
            anomaly .................................. 36
            commencement notification ................. 37
            extension ................................. 39
            remuneration ..............................41
```

maternity pay 79–113
    absence notification 91–4
    accounting records 104–5
    additional records 105
    agency workers 85–6
    allowance 79–82
    casual workers, seasonal/regular 79, 86–7
    contractual 96
    employer, change of 87–8, 96, 97
    employer insolvency 106
    mistakes 101–103
    pregnancy, types of 106–108
    qualifying week calculation 83
    records 103–5
    weekly earnings, average 83–4, 88–9, 91
    see also statutory maternity pay
maternity pay period
    (MPP) 97–98
    birth before commencement 98
    commencement, timing of 93, 97
    disentitlement 98–99
    employment termination after qualifying week 98
    payment and administration 99–101
    and premature birth 107
    statutory maternity pay (SMP) 95–6, 107
    working once commenced 97, 99
medical certificate/evidence 5, 50, 61, 80, 131, 136
medical evidence 83, 94, 104
Member States
    Directives 22
    maternity pay period (MPP) 97
miscarriages 106
mistakes and statutory maternity pay (SMP) 101–103
MPP *see* maternity pay period
multiple births 107

National Insurance Contributions
    (NIC) 101–102
    compensation 101–102, 117
    disputes and appeals 117
    maternity pay 80, 82, 83, 88, 91, 99, 103, 105
NDR *see* notified date of return

NIC *see* National Insurance Contributions
night work 131–2, 136
non-reinstatement other than redundancy 57–9
Northern Ireland Equal Opportunities Commission 51
notice *see* giving notice; notification
Notice of Appeal 120
notice payments 75
notification
    of date of return 49–50
    of intention to take maternity leave 36, 45
    late 46
    of maternity absence 91–4, 105
    requirement exceptions 92–3
notified date of return (NDR) 40, 50, 52, 53, 57, 71, 73–4

off-setting 100
Osborne v Thomas Bolton & Sons Ltd COIT 794/248 46
outside European Community (EC) 96, 97, 99

P11 *see* Deduction Working Sheets
P14 *see* End of Year Returns
P35 *see* Annual Statement, Declaration
and Certificate
"payday" 88, 123–4
PAYE 99, 101
payment 8–10
    and administration of statutory
        maternity pay (SMP) 99–101
    contractual 108
    entitlement during time off 8–10
    during maternity leave 34
    method 100
    refusal 12, 13
    week 9
    see also earnings; maternity pay;
        Statutory Sick Pay
period of interruption 52
"perks" 41, 48, 134
physical agents 128–30
pregnancy, types of 106
pregnant workers 62, 127, 130–3, 135

Pregnant Workers Directive 34, 127–132
    annex I 128–9
    annex II 130, 131
    Article 2 (definitions) 127–8
    Article 4 (assessment) 128–9
    Article 5 (adjust working conditions) 129–31
    Article 6 (specific risks) 131
    Article 7 (night work) 131–2
    Article 8 (maternity leave) 136
    assessment 128–9
    health and safety 134–5
    requirements 128–31
    state versus private sector employers 127
premature birth 37, 81, 107
protected period 24
qualifying week (QW) 83
    calculation 83
    employment termination 92
    maternity pay
        absence notification 91–4
        agency workers 85
        casual workers 87
        weekly earnings 83, 88–9, 90
    maternity pay period 88, 97
    premature birth 107
QW *see* qualifying week

reasonableness 62, 71
"reasonably practicable" 83, 92
    maternity leave notification 37
    return to work 46, 52
Reay v Sunderland Health Authority (unreported) 48
recently given birth 62, 127, 128, 131–3, 135
reclaiming statutory maternity pay (SMP) 101
records 103–105
    accounting 104
    additional 105
    wages 103
recovery of statutory maternity pay (SMP) 101
redundancy 69–77
    and alternative employment 70–1
    consultation 72, 74–5

during maternity leave	57
implementation	73–5
monies, repayment of	75
notice payments	75
and short-term maternity leave	72–3
and unreasonable refusal of offer	71

remuneration whilst suspended 134
return to work
    early 40
    notification of date 49–50, 75
    postponement 50–1, 52–3
    reinstatement 57–9
    right 42, 53–4, 71, 92
    see also intention to return; maternity leave;
      notified date of return
review as opposed to appeal 122–3
risks *see* specific risks
Ryan v Sporting Tours Promotions Ltd (unreported) 47

safety *see* health and safety
Secretary of State 116, 117, 121–2, 123, 125
self-employed 79, 80, 82
Sex Discrimination Act 1975 .... 19–21, 22, 27
    redundancy 75
    return to work 56
sex discrimination and pregnancy 19–31
    case law 20–2
    English approach v the European
      Community approach 22, 27–9
    Sex Discrimination Act 1975 .... 19–21, 22, 27
shift work *see* night work
short-term maternity leave and return to work 34–43
    absence prior to 11th week before expected
      week of confinement 38
    accrued right 35–6
    checklist 43
    commencement 36
    contractual rights 40–1, 42
    early return 40
    failure to return after 14th week 40
    intention to return notification 42
    leave duration 35, 38

```
            pregnancy notification ...................... 36-7
            redundancy after leave ..................... 70, 72
            redundancy during leave ...................... 42
            statutory maternity pay entitlement ............. 41
            versus long-term maternity leave .............. 34-5
sickness benefit ........................................ 82
*Sillars v Charringtons Fuels Ltd* (1989) ICR 475 ........... 86
small employers ................................. 57-8, 59
SMP *see* statutory maternity pay
SMP1 form ........................... 80, 96, 102, 103
            issued by mistake ........................ 102-103
SMP14 form ........................................... 117
Social Security
            Act 1986 ...................................... 79
            Appeal Tribunal ................... 117-19, 120, 122
            Commissioner ...................... 119, 120-1, 122
            Contributions and Benefits Act 1992 ............. 79
            *see also* Department of Social Security
specific risks (Article 6) ........................... 131
"specified reasons" ................................... 53
SSP *see* Statutory Sick Pay
statement, written .......................... 92, 115-6
statutory maternity pay (SMP) ............... 79, 82-109
            form SMP1 (non-entitlement) ....... 80, 96, 102-103
            form SMP14 (dispute) ......................... 117
            (General) Amendment Regulations 1990 ........ 86-7
            not payable ........................... 80, 88, 91
            return to work ................................ 41
            sex discrimination ............................ 29
            *see also* higher rate; lower rate
statutory records ............................... 103-105
Statutory Sick Pay (SSP) ....................... 99, 116
stillbirths ....................................... 106-107
"substantially less favourable" ....................... 133
suspension .................................. 59, 132-4
            of contract ................................ 48, 75


tax *see* income tax
test period ............................................ 80
time limit
            application to adjudication officer ............. 116
                query adjudication officer findings ........... 118
```

    formal decisions enforcement 123–5
    Social Security Commissioner 120
time off work see ante-natal care
Trade Union Reform and Employment Rights Act 1993
    ante-natal care 3
    health and safety 127–132
    maternity leave 33
    maternity pay 103
    redundancy 70, 72, 74
    return to work
        alternative employment 59
        dismissals 39, 58, 60–2
        long-term maternity leave 43, 50, 52, 53–5
    suspension rights 59
trade unions 119
Transfer of Undertakings (Protection
    of Employment) Regulations 1981 87
TURERA 1993 *see* Trade Union Reform and
    Employment Rights Act 1993
Turley v Allders Department Store (1980) ICR 66 20–1
twins 107

vacancy, suitable alternative 70–1
VDU *see* display screen equipment

wage records 105
Webb v EMO Air Cargo (UK) Ltd (1993) IRLR 272 .... 5–8, 35
    return to work 33–4
    sex discrimination 25, 26, 27, 28–9, 35, 40, 51
workers
    agency 85–6
    casual 79, 86–7
    see also breast-feeding; employees;
        pregnant; recently given birth
working
    conditions 128–32, 135
    during maternity pay period (MPP) 97, 99
    hours, normal 5–7, 9–10